PROLO YOUR BACK PAIN AWAY!

Dear family, friends, colleagues,
chronic pain sufferers, and athletes
hampered by injury,

Remember that no matter what happens
in life; no matter how bad the
pain gets — you can always

Prolo Your Pain Away!

Sincerely,

Ross & Marion

PROLO YOUR BACK PAIN AWAY!

Curing Chronic Back Pain with Prolotherapy

ROSS A. HAUSER, M.D.
Physical Medicine and Rehabilitation Specialist
and
MARION A. HAUSER, M.S., R.D.
Registered Dietitian and Nutritional Specialist

© BEULAH LAND PRESS ■ OAK PARK, ILLINOIS

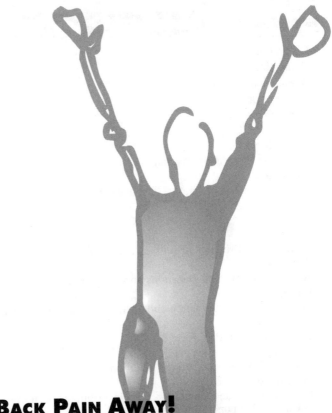

PROLO YOUR BACK PAIN AWAY!

ISBN 0-9661010-2-2

Text and illustrations copyright © 2000, Beulah Land Press
Cover and page design copyright © 2000
Illustrations and Charts by Thomas Penna, M. Hurley, Joe Faraci, Megan Barnard and Chris Athens

Published by Beulah Land Press
715 Lake Street, Suite 600, Oak Park, Illinois 60301

Printed in the United States of America

Design by Teknigrammaton Graphics
773-973-1614 • Teknigram@worldnet.att.net
7312 N. Hamilton • Chicago, IL 60645

TABLE OF CONTENTS

DISCLAIMER

The information presented in this book is based on the experiences of the authors, publishers, and editors, and is intended for informational and educational purposes only. In no way should this book be used as a substitute for your own physician's advice.

Because medicine is an ever-changing science, readers are encouraged to confirm the information contained herein with other sources. The authors, publishers, and editors of this work have used sources they believe to be reliable to substantiate the information provided. However, in view of the possibility of human error or changes in medical sciences, neither the authors, publishers, or editors, nor any other party who has been involved in the preparation or publication of this work warrants that the information contained herein is in every respect accurate or complete, and they are not responsible for any errors or omissions or for the results obtained from the use of such information. This is especially true, in particular, when an athlete or person in pain receives Prolotherapy and a bad result occurs. The authors, publishers, and editors of this book do not warrant that Prolotherapy is going to be effective in any medical condition and cannot guarantee or endorse any certain type of Prolotherapy, solution used, or practitioner. It is the responsibility of the individual athlete or person who receives Prolotherapy to thoroughly research the topic and pick a particular practitioner that they feel is qualified to perform the procedure. As of this writing there is no certification available in Prolotherapy training. Any licensed medical or osteopathic doctor in the United States can perform Prolotherapy according to the laws.

Physicians should use and apply the technique of Prolotherapy **only** after they have received extensive training and demonstrated the ability to safely administer the treatment. The author, publisher, editors, or any other person involved in this work, is not responsible if physicians who are unqualified in the use of Prolotherapy administer the treatment based solely on the contents of this book, or if they receive training but do not administer it safely and a bad result occurs.

If Prolotherapy or any other treatment regime described in this book appears to apply to your condition, the authors, publisher, and editors recommend that a formal evaluation be performed by a physician who is competent in treating pain and athletic injuries with Prolotherapy. Those desiring treatment should make medical decisions with the aid of a personal physician. No medical decisions should be made solely on the contents or recommendations made in this book.

1

Too many people give up on their dreams. One dream of ours and of many others involved is currently being fulfilled... to all the people helping fulfill the dream of **Beulah Land Natural Medicine Clinic** we dedicate this book. Beulah Land represents all that is good and pure in this life...

Beulah Land Natural Medicine Clinic at the time of the writing of this book is just a free Christian medical clinic that meets in the basement of The First Baptist Church of Thebes, Illinois on eight days out of each year. Yes, it is still a dream... to walk along Shawnee National Forest and to look as far as the eye can see—not sterile white buildings, but log cabins, trees, animals, ponds, and streams. Each day people receive prayer, song, massage, and other things to promote physical as well as spiritual healing. They are given the best natural treatments from around the world, all the while volunteers read from the Bible, with praise music in the background. We hope to have a recreational center with an Olympic sized pool, tennis courts, and exercise equipment, for volunteers and patients. Another hope is to have volunteer residence buildings where each volunteer family is given a suite with bedrooms, kitchen, and fireplace, all in a country setting.

The largest building, Beulah Land Natural Medicine Clinic, is hopefully going to be the first building built. It will be the outpatient center with a full IV/chelation center, 20 examination rooms, surgical suites, ozonated pool/Jacuzzi for patients, a full service laboratory, and procedure rooms. We hope to eventually have an on-site patient program, where people with chronic diseases such as cancer, rheumatoid arthritis, severe obesity, multiple sclerosis, progressive arthritis, and other chronic degenerative diseases can stay temporarily while they are being treated at the clinic. All of these services will be given free of charge. Since its inception, Beulah Land Natural Medicine Clinic has offered all services free of charge. This is the dream, the dream of Beulah Land...

Many are already helping fulfill the dream of Beulah Land. Forty-five acres of land has been purchased to build the first building. Steve and Daphene Huffman are the first full-time missionaries employed to help fulfill the dream. Marla Blakemore, Richard Boomer, Rodney Van Pelt, Pastor Carl Fisher, MaryLou Daguio, Ross and Marion Hauser make up the board given the monumental task of guiding Beulah Land and trying to raise the initial $2.0 million dollars to build the first completely free, comprehensive natural medicine clinic in the world! All of the board members also volunteer their time at each of the clinics.

To our many volunteers who help at each clinic including Mary Ellen Shlamer, Linda Fisher, Marge Cain, all of our staff at Caring Medical in Oak Park, and the doctors who close their practices to come and help us: Mark Wheaton, Bill Hambach, Kurt Ehling, Michelle Henry, and Rodney Van Pelt... thank you for your persistent, love, dedication, and hard work. The dream of Beulah Land will never be fulfilled unless others like you give so generously of their time. To our many donors thus far, as the Bible says "Be fruitful and multiply." Of course, to the greatest patients in the world—we love injecting you, and of course, we love talking with you! Thanks for your continued encouragement and for being so kind, even though we often do not quite get to you at your appointment time...you know we are giving you all that we have!

To all who are helping fulfill the dream of Beulah Land—this book is dedicated to you...

"But just as you excel in everything—in faith, in speech, in knowledge, in complete earnestness and in your love for us—see that you also excel in this grace of giving." 2 Corinthians 8:7

It is through your generosity and caring that Beulah Land Natural Medicine Clinic can offer the services of a natural medicine facility to those in need without charge.

Sincerely with warm regards,

Marion A. Hauser, MS, RD
Ross A. Hauser M.D.

Ross and Marion Hauser

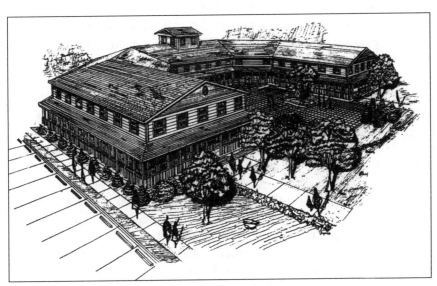

Artist's rendering of the proposed Beulah Land Clinic Building

ACKNOWLEDGEMENTS

L ife has been good to us. We have enjoyed the support of parents who always told us to "just do your best," and the love of a wonderful family, especially that of mom and dad Boomer, mom and dad Hauser, grandma and grandpa, Staci, Kyle, Alex, Torin, Ellen, Sara, Tommy, and Liz. Grandma, we cannot thank you enough for all you have taught us. We love you and miss you every day.

A pupil is only as wise as his teachers. We have had wonderful teachers along the way. Of course, none of the work in Prolotherapy would have been possible without Gustav A. Hemwall, M.D. Thank you Dr. Hemwall, for sharing your vast knowledge, and more importantly, what it means to be an "old fashioned" doctor. We miss you.

We would like to thank some of our colleagues who have shared their knowledge with us to help us learn more things to help people: Doug Kaufmann, Jean Liu, Gail Gelsinger, R.N., William Mauer, M.D., and Mike and Su Auberle, R.N. We owe a great debt to Steven Elsasser, M.D., who mentored us and started us on the vast search of finding ways to heal the body naturally, without pharmaceuticals. We are who we are, in part, because of the influence of our late pastor and his wife, Peter and Marla Blakemore, in our lives. We cannot begin to thank you for all of the things you have taught us. Pastor Peter, we look forward to seeing you in heaven. We still miss you every day. Marla, you are a great friend and confidant. Thank you for being there when we need you.

We have lost many loved ones along our journey through life. A day does not go by that we do not think of you: Grandma, Pastor Peter, Pastor John, Dr. Steve, Dr. Dave, Dr. Hemwall, and Larry. We look forward to the day when we will see you again in heaven.

Thank you to our new pastor, Ray Pritchard, and his wife Marlene. You have helped us to "keep believing," even through the tough times. Thank you to Calvary Memorial Church for making the message of Jesus Christ come alive!

What would we do without friends? We have been blessed with great friends: Don and Kristy; Marla and the kids; Tim, Sheila, and the kids; Steve and Candace; Larry and Mary; the gang at the Thursday night Bible study; and the whole clan at Harrison Street Bible church.

We have the greatest staff in the world at Caring Medical and Rehabilitation Services. To Tony, Brenda, Audrey, MaryLou, Teresa, Peter, Diane, Anne, Patsy, Walter, Cathy, Romona, Patti, Lisa, Nicole and Sandy: thank you for making work so enjoyable. Thank you for working so hard and going the extra mile. Thanks for giving so willingly of yourselves with hugs, listening ears, and tears to those who have walked through our doors with their many hurts and sorrows.

We also have great consultants who help us keep everything together. Nick, you were there with the first computer, and look at us now. Bill, thanks for helping us keep our business afloat. Thanks to our attorneys, David Hoy and Kirkpatrick Dilling, for all of your advice and counsel. Thanks to Jay and Bret for your willingness to help us. Thanks to Tim and Jack for making Caring Medical the facility it is today.

Thank you to Thomas Penna, for coming through in the clutches with your wonderful illustrations. Thank you to Joe Faraci for providing all of the initial illustrations. Thanks to Megan Barnard and Chris Athens for your creative illustrations.

Thank you to everyone at Kipland Publishing for helping to launch *Prolo Your Pain Away!* especially K.J., Cathy, and Tonya. Thank you to Molly for taking on this project and making it a huge *success*. Thank you to Event Management Services, especially Martha, Marsha, and Harriet, for helping us spread the word about Prolotherapy and sell out of the first printing in one year.

Thank you to the many volunteers who give of their time to Beulah Land Natural Medicine Clinic, especially Daphene and Steve Huffman; Mary Ellen Schlamer; Pastor Carl and Linda Fisher; Kim and Rodney Van Pelt, M.D.; Dick Boomer; Mark Wheaton, M.D.; Marge Cain; Brenda Lewis; Brodie Hackney; Rita Powelkop; Kurt Ehling, D.C., Bill Hambach, D.C., Grace Cole; Peter, Andrew, Gracelyn, Elizabeth, and Marla Blakemore; Michelle Henry, N.D.; Tim, Sheila, Heidi, and Heather Phillips; Eddie Bennett; and the rest of the wonderful volunteers from the First Baptist Church in Thebes, the folks from southern Illinois and southeast Missouri, and all of the other doctors and volunteers who help us when they can.

Thank you to Kurt Pottinger for your many hours spent putting *Prolo Your Pain Away!* together. You helped make it a best-seller!

Thank you to Barry Weiner from Media for Doctors for your undying support, your humor, your invaluable advice, your many, many hours of work, and most of all, your friendship. What would we do without you?

We especially want to thank Teresa Coconato for her countless hours of hard work, research, organization, dedication, patience, tenacity, and diligence with this project. We could not have done it without you. Thanks for the laughs when the going got tough!

I especially want to thank my wife and best friend for the many hours spent editing and writing this book. Thanks for getting us out of all of the fiascos I get us into and sticking by me no matter what. Thanks for changing your career and running our clinic together.

Ross, thanks for the ideas behind the books. I know I will never be out of a job! Thanks for the opportunity to work on these projects with you. Your diligence is amazing!

Finally, we want to thank the One who makes everything possible. Thank you God for the gift of grace and salvation. King David wrote several thousand years ago: "But as for me, I will always have hope; I will praise you more and more. My mouth will tell of your righteousness, of your salvation although I know not its measure. I will proclaim your righteousness, Yours alone."[1]

Our first book *Prolo Your Pain Away! Curing Chronic Pain with Prolotherapy* was released in October of 1997. We were not quite prepared for the response we received to our book. We not only sold all of our printed copies, but we were inundated with calls from chronic pain sufferers, as well as physicians wanting to learn more about this technique of Prolotherapy. This is what we had hoped to accomplish with the book: to make chronic pain sufferers aware of a curative technique that can help end their suffering.

The response to our second book, *Prolo Your Sports Injuries Away! Curing Sports Injuries and Enhancing Athletic Performance with Prolotherapy* has been even more overwhelming. The first book explained a new and different option for chronic pain sufferers: Prolotherapy. The chronic pain community was rattled a bit because of this. However, when you read the chapter in *Prolo Your Sports Injuries Away!* entitled, "The Twenty Myths of Sports Injuries" you will understand why the sports medicine industry was *and is* still shaking.

WHAT IS PROLOTHERAPY?

The primary concept that must be understood here is that the fundamental process by which the human body heals and strengthens is **inflammation**. The traditional philosophy of using some type of **anti-inflammatory** method such as rest, ice, elevation, compression, anti-inflammatory medications, or cortisone shots to heal injury is totally flawed. **No inflammation, no healing. It is that simple.**

The concept of Prolotherapy is radical compared to traditional treatments for chronic pain and sports injuries, yet it is so simple. Inject a mild irritant or proliferant at the site of the pain or injury to stimulate healing to the specific area. This concept is too basic for the highly intellectual scholars in the field of chronic pain management. Healing the multitude of chronic painful conditions with such a technique is unthinkable

Prolotherapy as defined by *Webster's Third New International Dictionary* is "the rehabilitation of an incompetent structure, such as a ligament or tendon, by the induced proliferation of cells." "Prolo" comes from the word proliferate (or grow). Prolotherapy injections proliferate or stimulate the growth of new, normal ligament and tendon tissue.

Prolotherapy is based on the concept that the cause of most chronic musculoskeletal pain is ligament and/or tendon weakness (or laxity). Ligaments connect the bones together to provide stability for the joints whereas; tendons connect muscles to the bone providing movement of the joints. When ligaments become weakened, the overlying muscles contract to stabilize the particular joints because the ligaments can no longer do their job. The result is muscle spasms and "knots."

Movement is painful because the tendons are weakened and the muscles are spasming. Stimulating the growth with Prolotherapy, thereby strengthening the ligaments and tendons, can relieve **most** chronic painful conditions.

In simple terms, Prolotherapy stimulates the body to repair painful areas. This is a good way to explain it to your friends, physicians, family, coaches, or trainers. The painful area is commonly a ligament(s) or tendon(s). Prolotherapy stimulates the body to repair this area. It does this by starting the normal healing mechanisms of the body. The injured athlete or chronic pain patient forms normal, healthy, strong tissue in the painful area after Prolotherapy has been administered, ridding the body of the abnormal, weak, painful tissue.

CONDITIONS TREATED WITH PROLOTHERAPY

When people read *Prolo Your Pain Away! Curing Chronic Pain with Prolotherapy,* they were amazed to find out the number of conditions that Prolotherapy could help. Often a person bought the book just to read the section about headaches or low back pain. They were unaware that Prolotherapy had been successful in eliminating many other painful conditions, such as the pain of arthritis, Fibromyalgia, herniated discs, degenerated discs, spondylolisthesis, migraines, RSD, TMJ, sciatica, tension headaches, osteoporosis, vulvodynia, coccydynia, loose joints, carpal tunnel syndrome, Morton's neuroma, myofascial pain, pregnancy back pain, cancer bone pain, and a host of other painful conditions.

When athletes read *Prolo Your Sports Injuries Away! Curing Sports Injuries and Enhancing Athletic Performance with Prolotherapy,* the same response was seen. Prolotherapy could be done on any ligament or joint of the body. Athletes began passing the word to their teammates that Prolotherapy could be used for ligament sprains, tendonitis, heel spurs, Osgood-Schlatter disease, loose joints, rotator cuff problems, ACL tears, and a host of other joint problems. The book discusses over twenty different sports explaining the typical injuries seen in the various sports and how Prolotherapy can cure the injuries and enhance athletic performance for each sport. Athletes who were told their careers were over went on to have stellar careers after Prolotherapy. We cannot tell you the number of people who have avoided arthroscopes, cortisone shots, another Motrin prescription, meniscal surgery, laminectomies, and a host of other surgical procedures because of these two books.

WHY WRITE THIS BOOK?

In talking with patients and other Prolotherapy enthusiasts, we found the need to write shorter "topical" books. Longer books overwhelm some people. We did our best to add some humor to the books to make them fun to read.

"It is not that difficult to find humorous things to talk about living with him!" Marion states. "Hey, what are you insinuating?" Ross says, adding, "You, know, honey bunch, you tend to do some funny things." Marion holds her ground, "Like what?" "Well, what about the time when you came to the office in your pajamas? Or the time you ripped open your suitcase and started flinging your underwear in the lobby at that hotel in Germany?" Ross asks. "Seems to me that these were all things that *you* did, not me!" Marion answers. "Boy, some people are sooo confused!"

Back to the topic at hand. Anyone with a desire to learn more about Prolotherapy is encouraged to read *Prolo Your Pain Away! Curing Chronic Pain with Prolotherapy* and *Prolo Your Sports Injuries Away! Curing Sports Injuries and Enhancing Athletic Performance with Prolotherapy* to understand the full scope of ailments and injuries that are successfully treated with Prolotherapy. We hope these shorter books will stimulate you to do what many chronic pain sufferers and supposedly washed-up athletes have found. Throw away the anti-inflammatory medications; forget the cortisone shots; and pass on the surgery. Realize that your body uses inflammation to heal. May you be one who runs away from the traditional methods of treating chronic pain and sports injuries. After reading this book, run to the local Prolotherapy physician. We suspect you will know why so many chronic pain sufferers and athletes are learning that the best MRI scan is not a big machine that makes noise, but the thumb of a Prolotherapist (**M**y **R**eproducibility **I**nstrument). MRIs and x-rays cannot diagnose the cause of pain. Only a physician or health care provider who understands ligament and tendon weakness (laxity) can do this. You must not anti-inflame your pain to stay, but inflame your pain away. We hope that you realize that the needle is mightier than the scalpel... There is a cure for chronic pain and sports injuries... and that cure is Prolotherapy.

Marion Hauser, MS, RD
Ross A. Hauser M.D.

Ross and Marion Hauser

An open mind is an important asset in medicine. There is far more we do not understand about the body than is written in all the collective libraries of the world...

Prolotherapy has achieved in its fifty years of practice many staunch supporters both as providers and recipients, but has not become a part of mainstream medical care. Why is this so? First of all, one has to look at how medical research is processed in the United States. Industry, government, hospitals and universities produce the vast majority of good scientific research. In order to maintain appropriate statistical significance, achieve the highest ethical standard, respect quality of human and animal life, the studies become extraordinarily expensive to operate. Thus to launch research at any of these institutions there must be appropriate funding. In the case of government it takes an executive decision or act of congress. Universities need grants. Industry sponsors research at institutions, government and their own facilities if there is potential profit. Unfortunately, Prolotherapy, which uses simple and readily available compounds, has never attracted pharmaceutical interest. Thus nationally organized research has not been initiated. On the other hand a fair amount of study into the field has been provided by individual clinicians with interest and commitment to Prolotherapy. Their research is underfunded and criticized for study design, lack of controls, and openness of data collection (not blinded). To me this is very understandable, since Prolotherapy in this context is provided as part of clinical practices. *In the trenches of reality, the doctor's office, the physician is thrust daily into situations where patients with intractable symptoms beg for help. In such situations it is difficult for clinicians to perform research with placebo controls and blindness, the standards of allopathic medicine.*

Prolotherapy has not made it into mainstream western medicine not just because of lack of funding, but also because few students are exposed to it during their formative years of career choice; medical school. Allopathic medical schools pride themselves on adherence to scientific methodology and tend to emphasize the science of medicine, not its clinical delivery. Prolotherapy, and other nonscientific but clinically useful pursuits, i.e. chiropractic, osteopathic, etc., are not even touched upon. Also problematic for the development of Prolotherapy is the traditional breakup of medicine into body parts and systems, such as orthopedics, pulmonary medicine, oncology. There is no one left with the responsibility of teaching or ministering to the soft-tissues. *Allopathic medicine's omission has allowed for many non-traditional fields to flourish.*

Allopathic medicine, the cornerstone of modern medicine, is predicated on the scientific method. Knowledge is gained in a step ladder fashion. Each new piece of the research puzzle defines one element of a question. Thus there is an organized pattern to the world's enigmas. Alternative Medicine, referred to as complementary medicine, accumulates its wisdom through empiricism—information gathered via trial and error. (Prolotherapy falls under the umbrella of complementary medicine because of empirical methodology of data collection.) The data collected has variability dependent on the skill and focus of the clinician. This lack of consistently reliable data has biased western medicine to avoid alternative/complementary medicine for the more predictable allopathic medicine. Unfortunately, potentially effective treatments go unrecognized, buried deep within alternative/complementary medicine.

A rebirth of interest in alternative/complementary medicine, kindled in part from western medicine's poor track record with preventative medicine, combined with general interest in healthy lifestyles, nutrition, and exercise has stimulated many allopathic physicians to visit the teachings of alternative/complementary medicine and to seek information they believe useful in their practice of medicine. In addition, some researchers have taken paradigms of alternative/complementary medicine and have begun challenging them with the scientific method. This melding of alternative/complementary medicine with the scientific method provides a yield of predictable information that is far more beneficial than either perspective operating alone. This marriage has already led to treatments now widely accepted in western medicine. (Some antibiotics and chemotherapy).

Prolotherapy has become increasingly popular over the past few years. Its popularity stems from success achieved in specific types of injury—most particularly ligament injury. It is theorized that injury to ligaments not only causes pain but abnormal mechanical performance of a joint. Ligaments are the supportive rubber bands that hold joints in place and allow them to maintain optimal mechanical advantage for muscular driven activities. When ligaments are torn or stretched, the mechanics of the joint are altered. This leads to direct and referred pain. Injections of irritants such as dextrose cause a localized inflammatory response that stimulates deposition of collagen which strengthens ligaments. This in a sense tightens the rubber band holding the motion segment (joint) together, improves joint performance, and both directly and indirectly decreases pain. Conditions reported to respond well to Prolotherapy include: Achilles tendon tears, tennis elbow, sacroiliac joint dysfunction, facet joint arthropathy as well as others.

Ten years ago I was skeptical regarding Prolotherapy—I had heard the testimonials and I had spoken to senior physicians. I thought it was professional mass confusion until I developed my own experience. I was surprised about positive and lasting results on selected patients. **In my practice today, I routinely utilize Prolotherapy for management of mechanical low back pain discomfort and various sports-related injuries.** The mechanical back pain patients typically present with long-standing pain refractory to interventions including multiple surgeries. Often mechanical components develop because disc disease with leg pain causes a limp, which leads to a pelvic shift, pulling on muscles and results in pain. Physical examination reveals pain palpable along the sacrum at midline and where sacrum joins the pelvis (SI joint). If I can touch the pain in the sacral region the pain is unlikely coming from lumbar discs which are deeper and further up the spine. If the patient fails to get better with osteopathic manipulation and shoe orthotics, which compensate for pelvic shift, we provide proliferative injections.

Prolotherapy is the only methodology I have ever utilized that demonstrates potential for significant benefit, yet has limited risk. This technique has been reserved for refractory patients that manage to find a proficient provider, but is most effective on sub-acute injuries. As a practitioner of Prolotherapy, I encourage athletes and chronic pain patients with chronic soft tissue injuries to consider Prolotherapy. ***Prolotherapy is a secret that needs to be discovered.***

Remember—keep an open mind!

Lloyd Saberski

Lloyd R, Saberski, M.D.
Former Medical Director,
Yale University School of Medicine
Center for Pain Management
New Haven, Connecticut

A Word From C. Everett Koop, M.D.

Prolotherapy is the name some people use for a type of medical intervention in musculoskeletal pain that causes a proliferation of collagen fibers such as those found in ligaments and tendons, as well as a shortening of those fibers. The "prolo" in Prolotherapy, therefore, comes from proliferative.

Other therapists have referred to this type of treatment as Sclerotherapy. "Sclera" comes from the Greek word "sklera," which means hard. Sclerotherapy, therefore, refers to the same type of medical intervention which produces a hardening of the tissues treated—just as described above in the proliferation of collagen fibers.

Not many physicians are aware of Prolotherapy, and even fewer are adept at this form of treatment. One wonders why that is so. In my opinion, it is because medical folks are skeptical and Prolotherapy, unless you have tried it and proven its worth, seems to be too easy a solution to a series of complicated problems that afflict the human body and have been notoriously difficult to treat by any other method. Another reason is the simplicity of the therapy: Injecting an irritant solution, which may be something as simple as glucose, at the junction of a ligament with a bone to produce the rather dramatic therapeutic benefits that follow. Another very practical reason is that many insurance companies do not pay for Prolotherapy, largely because their medical advisors do not understand it, have not practiced it, and therefore do not recommend it. Finally, Prolotherapy seems too simple a procedure for a very complicated series of musculoskeletal problems which affect huge numbers of patients. The reason why I consented to write the preface to this book is because I have been a patient who has benefitted from Prolotherapy. Having been so remarkably relieved of my chronic disabling pain, I began to use it on some of my patients—but more on that later.

When I was 40 years old, I was diagnosed in two separate neurological clinics as having intractable (incurable) pain. My comment was that I was too young to have intractable pain. It was by chance that I learned that Gustav A. Hemwall, M.D., a practitioner in the suburbs of Chicago, was an expert in Prolotherapy. When I asked him if he could cure my pain, he asked me to describe it. When I had done the best that I could, he replied, "There is no such pain. Do you mean a pain..." And then he continued to describe my pain much better than I could. When I said, "That's it exactly," he said, "I can fix you." To make a long story short, my intractable pain was not intractable and I was remarkably improved to the point where my pain ceased to be a problem. Much milder recurrences of that pain over the next 20 years were retreated the same way with equally beneficial results.

I was so impressed with what Dr. Hemwall had done for me that on several occasions, just to satisfy my curiosity, I watched him work in his clinic and witnessed the unbelievable variety of musculoskeletal problems he was able to treat successfully. Many of his patients were people who had been treated for years by all sorts of methods, including major surgery, some of which had left them worse off than they were before. Many of his patients had the lack of confidence in further treatment and the low expectations that folks inflicted with chronic pain frequently exhibit. Yet I saw so many of them cured that I could not help but become a "believer" in Prolotherapy.

I was a pediatric surgeon, and there are not many times when Prolotherapy is needed in children because they just don't suffer from the same relaxation of musculoskeletal connections that are so amenable to treatment by Prolotherapy. But I noticed frequently that the parents of my patients were having difficulty getting into their coats, or they walked with a limp, or they favored an arm. I would ask what the problem was and then, if it seemed suitable, offer my services in Prolotherapy at no expense, feeling that I was a pediatric surgeon and this was really not my line of work. The results I saw in those many patients were just as remarkable as was the relief I had received in the hands of Dr. Hemwall. I was so impressed with what Prolotherapy could do for musculoskeletal disease that I, at one time, thought that might be the way I would spend my years after formal retirement from the University of Pennsylvania. But the call of President Reagan to be Surgeon General of the United States interrupted any such plans.

The reader may wonder why, in spite of what I have said and what this book contains, there are still so many skeptics about Prolotherapy. I think it has to be admitted that those in the medical profession, once they have departed from their formal training and have established themselves in practice, are not the most open to innovative and new ideas. Let me give an example. About 15 years after I first met Dr. Hemwall and was treated by him for my lower extremity pain, I began to develop serious pain in my right shoulder girdle and upper arm. I was treated by neck traction, which made me worse, and after sleeping in an awkward position on an airplane to London, I woke up with my right arm paralyzed.

Because of the wonderful care I received at St. Bartholomew's Medical College Hospital, I began to have muscle twitching in my paralyzed arm within three weeks; by six weeks I could open a door and after three months I was back at the operating table. What I learned was that abnormal motion in the skeletal system can produce both sensory and motor symptoms. I had both in my shoulder and arm. I was treated in London by cervical traction, but not as I had been in the United States—just pulling my neck off my shoulders by means of a sling under my chin and my skull—but I was treated by cervical traction with my head flexed forward and turned to one side. That relieved the pressure on the nerves involved which led to my recovery.

When I would have minor symptoms of the same type, I learned from my physiotherapy colleagues in London that the head weighs about 12 pounds and can be used as a means of cervical traction by lying prone on a bed with your shoulders at the edge of a mattress, letting your head hang forward (flexion), and turning it to the side of your pain. There were days that I could barely get my wallet out of my back pocket. I would have to "walk" my fingers across my hip to my pocket and then slowly extricate the wallet. That was my right hand into my right rear pocket. After five minutes of the previously described traction over the edge of a bed, I could put my right arm completely around my back to the other flank.

I was so impressed with what I had learned that, one day, while with a few of my orthopedic and neurosurgical colleagues, I demonstrated the improvement after hanging my head over a gurney outside the operating room. Instead of being impressed, they all walked away as skeptics, some of them thinking that I had faked the whole thing to impress them.

Prolotherapy is not a cure-all for all pain. Therefore, the diagnosis must be made accurately and the therapy must be done by someone who knows what he or she is doing. The nice thing about Prolotherapy, if properly done, is that it cannot do any harm. How could placing a little sugar-water at the junction of a ligament with a bone be harmful to a patient?

I hope that Dr. Hauser's book, written for laymen, will push them to inquire more about Prolotherapy and that it might receive the place in modern therapeutics that I think it really deserves.

C. Everett Koop, M.D., Sc.D.
Former United States Surgeon General

CHAPTER 1

My Story: What is a "Physiatrist?"

I was born on September 14, 1962.... Just joking! You have to learn to relax! Did you know that when we were children we laughed 80 times per day, but as adults we chuckle a measly 15 times per day?! This is especially significant because we do so many funny things.

While attending the University of Illinois Medical School, I had a difficult time deciding on an area of specialization. Family medicine seemed appealing, but working in the intensive care unit was not for me. Then a friend of mine, Steve Primack, now an attending radiologist at the University of Oregon, gave me a book that contained a comprehensive list of medical specialties. After reviewing it and praying with my wife about our future, I decided to look into the field of Physical Medicine and Rehabilitation.

Physical Medicine and Rehabilitation is a medical discipline approved by the American Board of Medical Specialties. After World War II, many soldiers returned home with disabilities, including amputations and spinal cord injuries. Previously, these veterans would have died from infection, but due to the discovery of penicillin they survived their injuries. Unfortunately, physicians had not been trained to care for those suffering from such disabilities. Out of this need eventually came the field of Physical Medicine and Rehabilitation, or Physiatry.

PHYSIATRY

A doctor who specializes in Physical Medicine and Rehabilitation is called a Physiatrist (pronounced *fizz-ee-at-trist*). No, I'm not a Psychiatrist. Look again. Physiatrist. Currently, there are approximately 5,000 board-certified Physiatrists in the United States. Physiatry requires four years of residency training after medical school. Rotations in stroke, multiple sclerosis, traumatic brain injury, amputations, cardiac rehabilitation, electromyography (EMG), spinal cord injury, neurology, sports medicine, orthopedic rehabilitation, and, of course, both acute and chronic pain management are all part of the residency program.

Physiatrists care for patients who suffer from a chronic or acute disease that has affected their ability to enjoy life and perform daily functions. A stroke victim, for example, requires medical attention as well as rehabilitation. Difficulties in blood pressure control, urination, speech, and swallowing are common problems that result from a stroke. Rehabilitation helps the patient relearn how to walk, talk, and live life.

Unfortunately, most people do not consult a Physiatrist because they do not know the profession exists. Even many Family Practice Physicians and Internists are unaware of Physiatry which is probably due to the fact that a rotation in Physical Medicine and Rehabilitation is not mandatory in medical schools. Physiatry is one medical field where a shortage of doctors exists. As man's life-span increases and more people survive disabling diseases, more Physiatrists will be needed.

WHERE IT ALL STARTED

I became fascinated with pain during my Physical Medicine residency. I began accumulating articles on bizarre pain syndromes and obtained quite a collection. (Everyone needs a hobby, right?) What struck me most was the magnitude of the pain problem. It seemed as though everyone either had pain themselves or knew someone who was suffering from chronic pain. I also saw the lack of significant pain relief by modern treatments such as surgery, physical therapy, and anti-inflammatory drugs.

It appeared that the longer people had pain, the less likely such treatments were going to help cure their chronic pain. Pain clinics and pain programs do help some people, but have a poor cure rate. Pain programs teach people to live with their pain. The psychological aspect of the pain is addressed, but in many cases the cause is not determined.

When I began seeing pain patients during my residency training program in Physical Medicine and Rehabilitation, I thought they were a very difficult group of people to treat. They often appeared depressed, and traditional approaches to pain management did not seem to help. Then I said to myself, "How would I feel if I had pain day after day and no one could find a cure?" The families of many who suffer from pain often begin doubting the reality of their loved one's pain. Many chronic pain patients who frequent pain clinics experience broken homes and lose their jobs because of the pain. It became evident to me that these patients' pain was indeed real and that pain pills and support groups did not cure the pain.

NATURAL MEDICINE

Then came Natural Medicine. I began learning about Natural Medicine the day I married Marion, a dietitian, on December 20, 1986. I watched as my life and sur-roundings slowly changed. Not long after we moved her things into our condo-minium, (After we were married—we're old fashioned, what can I say?), Marion axed fast-food from my diet. I have not eaten a can of Spaghetti-O's since our wed-ding. What sacrifices I have made! Marion introduced me to good-tasting spinach and drastically altered my diet. The chronic fatigue that I thought was from the intensity of medical training began to subside. I guess the rest is history!

Natural Medicine employs natural substances such as organic foods, herbs, vitamins, and minerals, as well as rest, exercise, and attention to faith in God to maintain and restore health. I began to see that modern medicine was not a cure-all for chronic diseases. Its lack of healing ability was especially evident as it per-tained to chronic disabling conditions caused by pain, multiple sclerosis, rheuma-toid arthritis, and cancer. I knew there had to be something to help all these suf-fering people.

One of my instructors, Oleh Paly, M.D., gave me a book by Linus Pauling, M.D., on the use of vitamin C in disease. He also directed me to various resources and organizations that specialize in natural healing techniques. This was my first real taste of Natural Medicine.

Soon after, I found myself taking acupuncture lessons and reading up on natural healing techniques. I tried the techniques on my wife. (After I have learned a technique, she always wants to be the first patient.) Since she survived, I tried them out on a few friends. (Most of them are still friends.) A friend from church, Mrs. Wright, was experiencing terrible pain. I tried all the treatment modalities and gizmos I knew of, but without success. Mrs. Wright eventually received treatment from Gustav A. Hemwall, M.D., the world's most experienced Prolotherapist. The Prolotherapy she received in her shoulder gave her a significant amount of relief. Mrs. Wright then encouraged me to learn about Dr. Hemwall's treatment.

PROLOTHERAPY

In April 1992, I contacted Dr. Hemwall and he allowed me to observe him in his clinic. I was astonished to see him perform 30, 50, or 100 injections on a patient at one time! He called his treatment Prolotherapy. The only other time I had come across the term was when a fellow resident showed me a book on the treatment. I later discovered that Dr. Hemwall was one of the authors of that book!

During the next few months, I spent a considerable amount of time in Dr. Hemwall's office. People traveled from all over the world to be treated by this 84-year-old man. I have nothing against age, but to think that someone would travel from places like England, Mexico, Florida, and California to receive pain management was incredible. I learned that if someone suffers from pain and someone else has a technique that will help alleviate the pain, time and expense are minor considerations.

It was clear that Dr. Hemwall was helping those whom traditional medicine had not helped. His average patient had been in pain for years and had tried it all: surgery, pain pills, anti-inflammatory medication, exercise, therapy, acupuncture, and hypnotism. Most patients had seen more than five physicians before consulting Dr. Hemwall. Almost all the patients I observed improved after one or two Prolotherapy treatments. People found relief from pain that had plagued them for years. Many said they wished they had known about Prolotherapy years ago.

Three months later, I began utilizing Prolotherapy in my medical practice as a treatment of chronic pain. I have effectively used Prolotherapy in nearly every joint of the body. In January 1993, I began working alongside Dr. Hemwall in his Prolotherapy practice. Since then, my wife and I have opened Caring Medical and Rehabilitation Services, S.C., a Natural Medicine Clinic that cares for people with chronic diseases using natural methods including Prolotherapy.

Since learning Prolotherapy, the practice of medicine has become more enjoyable. Prolotherapy has enabled us to offer a treatment that eliminates long-standing pain. Chronic pain, like cancer, sucks the lifeblood out of a person. It can disrupt families and lead them into bankruptcy if the pain prohibits the patient from holding a job. What a joy it will be when you or your loved ones find pain relief. We believe this book will lead you, or someone you know, down the path to healing chronic pain naturally with Prolotherapy. ■

CHAPTER 2

Introduction: The Technique and Its History

N othing was worse than a chronic low back pain patient walking into my office," said Gustav A. Hemwall, M.D., the world's most experienced Prolotherapist. "I would try exercise, corsets, and surgery, but nothing really helped."

In 1955, when Dr. Hemwall visited a scientific exhibit at the national meeting of the American Medical Association, that all changed. Recalling the meeting, Dr. Hemwall said, "At one particular exhibit I noticed a crowd of doctors listening to a doctor say he had a cure for low back pain. This fellow had written a book on it as well." That fellow was George S. Hackett, M.D., the father of Prolotherapy. **(See Appendix E, George S. Hackett AMA Presentations.)**

Once the crowd diminished, Dr. Hemwall asked Dr. Hackett how he could learn the treatment described in his book. Dr. Hackett responded by inviting Dr. Hemwall to observe him administering Prolotherapy. Dr. Hemwall became so proficient at administering the technique that Dr. Hackett would later refer patients to him. **(See Figure 2-1.)**

Dr. Hemwall remembers, "When I returned from that meeting, I quickly read Dr. Hackett's book describing Prolotherapy and treated my first patient. After a few sessions of Prolotherapy, this patient, instead of coming into the office in a wheel-chair, ran to catch four buses. From that point on, instead of dreading patients with low back pain, I began to look for them." That was 40 years ago. Since that time, some 10,000 patients have received Prolotherapy from Dr. Hemwall.

PROLOTHERAPY CASE REPORTS

Chronic low back pain management has taken a drastic turn from when the American Medical Association presented Dr. Hackett's Prolotherapy work at their national meetings in 1955. Now Prolotherapy is not covered in its journal and is rarely mentioned at national meetings. Unfortunately, for the millions of Americans suffering from chronic back and body pain, several events have led to the reduction in the number of physicians using Prolotherapy.

On August 8, 1959, the *Journal of the American Medical Association* reported a fatality after a Prolotherapy injection series. In the case report, Richard Schneider, M.D., wrote, "...in the instance reported here, it must be emphasized that the sclerosing solution [Prolotherapy solution] was not the usual sodium salt of the vegetable oil fatty acid as described in the original monograph [by Dr. Hackett], but instead a solution of zinc sulfate in 2.5 percent phenol."[1]

This physician also apparently injected this solution into the spinal canal, not at the fibro-osseous junction where ligaments and tendons attach to bone. Dr. Schneider ended the case report with, "...this technique of precipitating fibro-

GEORGE S. HACKETT. M. D.
616 FIRST NATIONAL BANK BUILDING
CANTON 2. OHIO

Jan. 25, 1957

Mrs. Lloyd D. Anderson
315 South 12th Street
Albia, Iowa

Dear Mrs. Anderson:

In reply to your letter of the 21st,
I would suggest that you consult: -

Gustav A. Hemwall, M.D.
839 North Central Avenue
Chicago, Illinois.

Dr. Hemwall is the only man that I
know of in your part of the country who is
experienced with this technic of treatment.
He was out here on several occasions and was
instructed in the technic by me, and I can
recommend him highly.

As to whether your condition could
be benefitted by this procedure, it is
impossible to give you any answer without
first having examined you to determine your
disability.

If I can be of further service,
please feel free to call on me.

Sincerely,

George S. Hackett, M.D.

Figure 2-1

osseous proliferation appears to be neither sound nor without extreme danger." It should be noted that the article was written by several physicians from the Neurosurgery department at the University of Michigan Hospital.

This tragic case occurred because the physician used too strong a proliferant and did not follow a cardinal rule of Prolotherapy: Prolotherapy injections are given only when the needle is touching the bone at the fibro-osseous junction, with the only exception being joint injections. Unfortunately, early Prolotherapy physicians did not follow Dr. Hackett's technique. The flawed method these physicians utilized caused some harmful effects and discouraged other physicians from administering Prolotherapy. When properly administered, Prolotherapy has no side effects and is effective in eliminating chronic pain.

PROLOTHERAPY SOLUTIONS

In his 19 years of using Sylnasol, a sodium salt of fatty acids and vegetable oil, Dr. Hackett observed no side effects. Dr. Hemwall noted that a number of years after Dr. Hackett's original work was published, Sylnasol was taken off the market due to a lack of demand. After several years of using various solutions, Dr. Hemwall found that a simple Dextrose and Lidocaine solution was the ideal proliferant. It produced only a small amount of pain following the procedure, yet resulted in complete pain relief after only a few treatments. More Dextrose solution could also be injected at one time than with the Sylnasol, allowing more areas of the body to be treated per visit.

Only recently has modern medicine figured out what Dr. Hemwall knew some 35 years ago: that a simple Dextrose solution is all that is needed to eliminate pain. Min-Young Kim, M.D., and associates from Yonsei University Medical College in Seoul, South Korea, studied 64 patients with chronic pain. Dr. Kim compared using a five percent Dextrose solution with the current standard trigger point injection solution of 0.5 percent Lidocaine and placebo. The study found that not only did the Dextrose solution prove to give statistically significant pain relief ($P<.01$) against placebo, it was that much better when compared to the Lidocaine solution. The study also found that in follow-up, the pain relief with the Dextrose solution remained. [2, 3]

The Prolotherapy solution used at Caring Medical and Rehabilitation Services is 15.0 percent Dextrose, 10.0 percent Sarapin, and 0.2 percent Lidocaine. Dr. Hemwall used the same solution without the Sarapin. The Dextrose is a corn extract and makes the solution more concentrated than blood (hypertonic), acting as a strong proliferant. Sarapin is used to treat nerve irritation and, in my experience, acts as a proliferant. Sarapin is an extract of the pitcher plant and is one of the few materials listed in the *Physician's Desk Reference* that has no known side effects. Lidocaine is an anesthetic that helps reinforce the diagnosis because the patient will experience immediate pain relief after the Prolotherapy injections.

The current Prolotherapy technique described in this book using these solutions has been administered by Dr. Hemwall and myself to more than 12,000 patients, in more than 40,000 treatment sessions, with more than four million injections given. Not one case of permanent nerve injury, paralysis, or death has been documented. The main side effect has been one to two days of soreness and stiffness after the procedure. This is not only from inflammation caused by the Prolotherapy injections, but occurs because the needle pierces the muscle to reach the fibro-osseous junction of the ligaments and tendons being treated.

The Dextrose solution, in addition to being safe, will not affect a diabetic's blood sugar level. If a patient is corn intolerant, other proliferant agents can be used. Such agents include sodium morrhuate (an extract of cod liver oil), preservative-free zinc sulfate, manganese, pumice, or a Dextrose-glycerine-phenol solution known as P2G. Incidentally, P2G was the proliferant used in the two double-blind studies that will be described in Chapter Four. [4,5]

MYOFASCIAL PAIN THEORY

In the early 1960's, after the damaging report in the *Journal of the American Medical Association,* Janet Travell, M.D., Internist, developed a treatment program for what she termed "Myofascial Pain Syndrome." She noted that patients with chronic pain had tight muscles and after the muscles were stretched or relaxed the pain would diminish. She also described trigger points or areas where muscle is tender to palpation. These trigger points refer pain to other areas of the body. She described these referral pain patterns in detail. [6]

Dr. Travell was an outstanding physician and gave successful care to then Senator John F. Kennedy five years prior to his presidential election. This led to her promotion to White House physician under President Kennedy and President Lyndon B. Johnson. Needless to say, her myofascial pain theory received a great deal of publicity and is embraced today as the main theory for chronic pain management.

Upon examination, the referral pain patterns laid out by Dr. Hackett in 1956 for ligament laxity are strikingly similar to the referral pain patterns described for muscles by Dr. Travell many years later. **(See Figure 2-2 to 2-5.)** The similarity exists because of the relationship between ligament laxity and muscle tenseness. Ligament weakness causes laxity or looseness in a joint. To stabilize the joint, the muscles tighten up. The overlying muscle is then overworked in an attempt to stabilize the loosened joint. This tense muscle produces trigger points or "knots."

Clinicians who use myofascial stretching techniques for tight muscles often find that the chronic pain is relieved temporarily but returns with the same intensity at some point after treatment. Myofascial therapy often only treats a symptom of the ligament weakness and, because the underlying ligament weakness is not dealt with, pain returns. Prolotherapy, by causing the growth of ligament tissue, treats the root cause of myofascial pain. By strengthening the ligaments, the joint

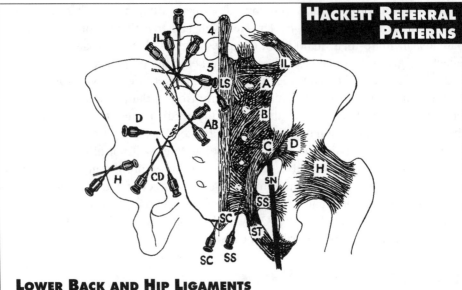

HACKETT REFERRAL PATTERNS

LOWER BACK AND HIP LIGAMENTS
TRIGGER POINTS OF LIGAMENTS

IL:	ILIOLUMBAR	ST:	SACROTUBEROUS
LS:	LUMBOSACRAL—SUPRA AND INTERSPINUS	SC:	SACROCOCCYGEAL
A, B, C, D:	POSTERIOR SACROILIAC	H:	HIP—ARTICULAR
SS:	SACROSPINUS	SN:	SCIATIC NERVE

Figure 2-2: Hackett Referral Patterns
Ligamentous structures of the lower back and hip that refer pain down the lower leg. The illustration shows the trigger points of pain and the needles in position for confirmation of the diagnosis and for treatment of ligament relaxation of the lumbosacral and pelvic joints.

stabilizes, so the muscles have no need to tighten. It is only then that trigger points and muscle tenderness are permanently eliminated.

CAT Scans, MRI Scans, and X-Rays

The next reason for the diminished use of Prolotherapy was the invention of the computerized axial tomography (CAT) scan. The CAT scan became widely available in the early 1970's and was used, among other things, to view the inter-vertebral disc. Chronic pain physicians in the early 1970's found abnormalities in this area and concluded that the disc problems caused chronic pain. Millions of people underwent surgical procedures to correct some "abnormality" of the disc as seen on the CAT scan, only to experience minimal pain relief.

Not until the early 1980's were the CAT scans of people without pain exam-ined.[7] A study published in 1984 by Sam W. Wiesel, M.D., found that 35 percent of the population, irrespective of age, had abnormal findings on CAT scans of their lower backs even though they had no pain complaints. In CAT scans of peo-ple over 40 years of age, 50 percent had abnormal findings. Twenty-nine percent

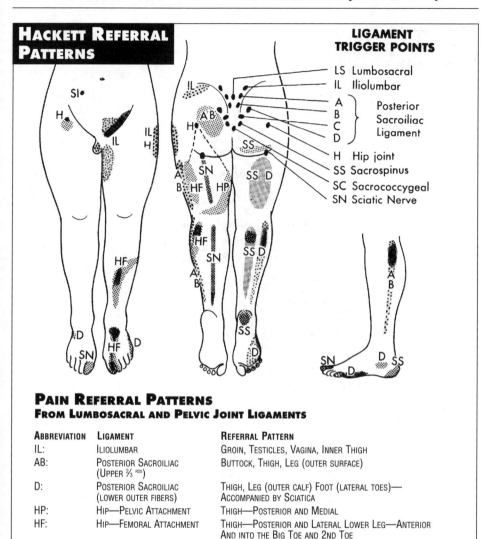

HACKETT REFERRAL PATTERNS

LIGAMENT TRIGGER POINTS

LS Lumbosacral
IL Iliolumbar
A ⎫
B ⎬ Posterior
C ⎪ Sacroiliac
D ⎭ Ligament
H Hip joint
SS Sacrospinus
SC Sacrococcygeal
SN Sciatic Nerve

PAIN REFERRAL PATTERNS
FROM LUMBOSACRAL AND PELVIC JOINT LIGAMENTS

ABBREVIATION	LIGAMENT	REFERRAL PATTERN
IL:	ILIOLUMBAR	GROIN, TESTICLES, VAGINA, INNER THIGH
AB:	POSTERIOR SACROILIAC (UPPER ⅔ RDS)	BUTTOCK, THIGH, LEG (OUTER SURFACE)
D:	POSTERIOR SACROILIAC (LOWER OUTER FIBERS)	THIGH, LEG (OUTER CALF) FOOT (LATERAL TOES)— ACCOMPANIED BY SCIATICA
HP:	HIP—PELVIC ATTACHMENT	THIGH—POSTERIOR AND MEDIAL
HF:	HIP—FEMORAL ATTACHMENT	THIGH—POSTERIOR AND LATERAL LOWER LEG—ANTERIOR AND INTO THE BIG TOE AND 2ND TOE
SS:	SACROSPINUS & SACROTUBERUS	THIGH—POSTERIOR LOWER LEG—POSTERIOR TO THE HEEL
SN:	SCIATIC NERVE	CAN RADIATE PAIN DOWN THE LEG

Figure 2-3: Hackett Referral Patterns
Ligament referral pain patterns from structures in **Figure 2-2.**

showed evidence of herniated discs, 81 percent facet degeneration (arthritis), and 48 percent lumbar stenosis (another form of arthritis). In other words, for people over 40 years of age who do not have symptoms of pain, a 50 percent chance of abnormality on their CAT scans exists, including a herniated disc.

In regard to pain management, diagnostic tests such as x-rays, magnetic resonance imaging (MRI) scans, or CAT scans should never take the place of a listening ear and a strong thumb to diagnose the cause of chronic pain. It is necessary for the clinician to understand where the pain originates and radiates. In other

HACKETT REFERRAL PATTERNS

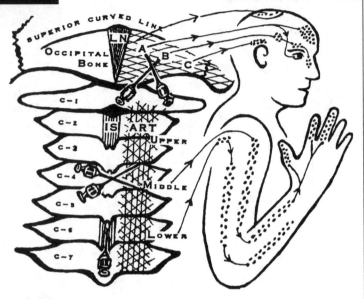

HEAD AND NECK REFERRAL PAIN PATTERNS
LIGAMENT AND TENDON RELAXATION

AREA OF WEAKNESS	REFERRAL PATTERN
OCCIPUT AREA A	FOREHEAD AND EYE
OCCIPUT AREA B	TEMPLE, EYEBROW AND NOSE
OCCIPUT AREA C	ABOVE THE EAR
CERVICAL VERTEBRAE #1-#3 (UPPER)	BACK OF NECK AND POSTERIOR SCAPULAR REGION (NOT SHOWN)
CERVICAL VERTEBRAE #4-#5 (MIDDLE)	LATERAL ARM AND FOREARM INTO THE THUMB, INDEX AND MIDDLE FINGER
CERVICAL VERTEBRAE #6-#7 (LOWER)	MEDIAL ARM AND FOREARM INTO THE LATERAL HAND, RING AND LITTLE FINGER

Figure 2-4: Hackett Referral Patterns
Head and neck ligament referral pain patterns.

words, what is the referral pattern? Unfortunately, most physicians do not know the referral patterns of the ligaments, as seen in **Figures 2-2, 3, 4, 5.** In summary, it should be obvious that an x-ray should not be used solely as the criterion for determining the cause of a person's pain.

To properly diagnose the cause of a person's pain it is important for the physician to touch the patient. Medical doctors are too quick to prescribe an anti-inflammatory medication or order an MRI. The best MRI scan is a physician's thumb, which we call **My R**eproducibility **I**nstrument, used to palpate the ligament or tendon suspected to be the problem. If the diagnosis is correct, a positive "jump sign" will occur because the weakened ligament or tendon will be very tender to palpation. If the physician does not reproduce a person's pain during an examination, the

GLUTEUS MEDIUS MUSCLE
REFERRAL PATTERN
JANET TRAVELL, M.D.

THE GLUTEUS MEDIUS MUSCLE REFERS PAIN DOWN THE LATERAL LEG AND INTO THE BUTTOCK REGION.

HIP LIGAMENT
REFERRAL PATTERN
GEORGE S. HACKETT, M.D.

THE HIP LIGAMENTS ALSO REFER PAIN DOWN THE LATERAL LEG AND INTO THE BUTTOCK REGION.

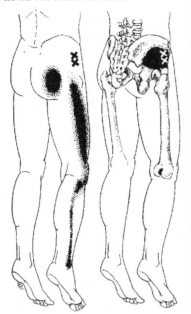
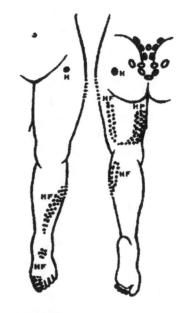

Figure 2-5: Comparison of Travell and Hackett Referral Patterns
Notice the similarities between the referral patterns.

Left: illustration: Travell—*Myofacial Pain and Dysfunction: The Trigger Point Manual*, Vol. 1, 2nd Ed., © Janet Travell, M.D. Used with permission.

likelihood of eliminating the pain is slim. How can a physician make a correct diagnosis without reproducing the pain? Our patients often say that this initial examination was the first real examination they have had for their pain.

It is not uncommon for a patient to leave our office after the initial consultation, before beginning Prolotherapy treatments, keenly aware of their pain source area. When patients confront Ross with this, he always smiles and says, "What did you expect? You came to a pain doctor!" The point is, a physician must reproduce the pain in order to document the exact pain-producing structure. Once this is located, Prolotherapy injections to strengthen the area will likely eliminate the pain.

THE INSPIRATION FOR THIS BOOK

Our inspiration to fulfill our dreams of writing these books about Prolotherapy came in the summer of 1995 when we visited Cornerstone to Health, a Natural Medicine clinic operated by Gail Gelsinger, R.N. Dr. Hauser examined 18 of the clinic's patients who, despite being on a good nutrition program, continued to suffer from chronic pain, and successfully treated each patient with Prolotherapy.

When we returned a few months later, twice as many patients desired Prolotherapy treatments. Unfortunately, our schedule prevents us from returning. As a result, a myriad of people needlessly suffer from chronic pain because the treatment of Prolotherapy is unavailable. We then realized how people could benefit from books about treating chronic pain with Prolotherapy.

Another reason for writing this book is to carry on where Dr. Hemwall has left off. In June 1996, Dr. Hemwall, at the age of 88, retired after 60 years of practicing medicine and 40 years of administering Prolotherapy. Because Dr. Hemwall had the privilege of learning Prolotherapy from its originator, the more books that share his knowledge, the better.

During the 40 years that Dr. Hemwall administered Prolotherapy, he treated more than 10,000 chronic pain patients. One of those 10,000 patients said his pain "originated in my spine, went down across my inguinal ligament, down the inside of my thigh, skipped my knee, went down the inside of my calves, skipped my ankle, and came out the dorsum of my foot like a burn." The patient was describing a sacroiliac referral pattern, and Prolotherapy to the sacroiliac joint very effectively eliminated the pain. This patient would later become the Surgeon General of the United States, C. Everett Koop, M.D.

Dr. Koop says, "I personally know the benefits of Prolotherapy. I had intractable back pain which traveled down my leg. I received Prolotherapy to my back by Dr. Hemwall. After a few treatments, it [the pain] was gone. Seeing the benefits of Prolotherapy on myself, I used the technique on the parents of my patients. I was a pediatric surgeon. When I saw the parents of my patients limping or having trouble taking off their coats, I would offer to treat them with Prolotherapy. I did it all pro bono. Prolotherapy does remarkably well at eliminating the pain caused by ligament relaxation or weakness. For someone experienced in the technique, it is extremely safe and effective. I utilized the technique of Prolotherapy from 1960 to 1980 and found it extremely effective in eliminating the chronic pain that comes from ligament relaxation." [8]

For the past 25 years, Dr. Hemwall had been the main proponent and teacher of Prolotherapy in the United States. He was responsible for training more physicians and treating more people with Prolotherapy than anyone else. Without his perseverance, the Hackett technique of Prolotherapy may have vanished. We have been blessed to have worked under Dr. Hemwall as students, with him as partners, and beside him as colleagues. In this book, we hope to disseminate what we have gleaned from a man we very much admire.

THE WEAKNESS OF MODERN MEDICINE

While a wonderful and effective procedure known as Prolotherapy has been achieving pain relief for more than 50 years, modern medicine continues to search for drugs, devices, and surgical procedures to eliminate chronic pain. Anti-inflammatory drugs have become a multi-billion dollar business. While these drugs provide temporary relief, they do not correct the underlying condition causing the pain. Migraine headaches are not caused by an Ibuprofen deficiency. When these drugs do not give permanent relief, the next step is typically exercise or physical therapy. As with the drugs, physical therapy and exercise provide temporary relief for the pain during the therapy, but the pain often returns once the therapy concludes.

The next step down the wrong path for the chronic pain patient is a referral to a surgeon. Unfortunately for many, surgery has not been the promised end to their pain and often makes the problem worse. Surgeons often use x-ray technology as a diagnostic tool. This is often not appropriate to properly diagnose the pain source. It is not uncommon for an x-ray to reveal terrible arthritis in someone who experiences no symptoms, whereas an x-ray of someone who has terrible pain symptoms may reveal nothing.

After examining these x-rays, a surgeon may decide to remove a disc or cartilage tissue in an attempt to alleviate pain. The two questions to ask are: Who put that tissue there? For what purpose? God placed disc tissue there to stabilize and cushion the lower back, and cartilage tissue in the joints so that bones glide smoothly over one another. What happens when the disc and cartilage tissue are removed? If the disc is removed, the vertebral levels above and below the surgerized segment develop proliferative arthritis. This happens because these segments have to carry more of the force than they were designed to carry in the lower back. If the cartilage is removed, the bones no longer glide smoothly over one another. Soon after this, a person notices a crunching of the joint where the cartilage was removed. This crunching sound is arthritis. The end result of surgical procedures that remove cartilage, ligaments, and bone from knees, backs, and necks is often arthritis.

Unfortunately, medicine has lost the art of clinical diagnosis without the aid of fancy tests and machines. Prolotherapists (physicians who practice Prolotherapy) are trained to reproduce and effectively treat a painful area without the need for x-rays or expensive tests.

PROLOTHERAPY AS PAIN MANAGEMENT

Other unnatural, ineffective, and/or destructive means to relieve pain include the implantation of a spinal cord stimulator, botulism toxin injections into muscles, and radio frequency thermocoagulation of nerves and other bodily structures. These treatments sound impressive but end up changing or destroying God-given anatomy or other bodily processes often without a long-term cure of the painful condition. Chronic pain is not due to a spinal cord stimulator or botulism toxin deficiency. A more sensible, natural approach to pain management would be to repair the damaged and weakened tissue. Chronic pain is almost always due to weakened, damaged tissue. A herniated disc, for example, is better treated by allowing the regrowth of ligament tissue through which the disc herniated, than by removing the disc.

Nathaniel W. Boyd's book, *Stay Out of the Hospital*, describes ligament relaxation. "Once forcibly stretched by trauma, ligamentous tissue is unable to snap back to its original length. This being the case, it should not be very difficult to understand how the ligaments of any joint, once over-stretched, will leave the joint wobbly, loose, and unstable. Along with this instability very often comes chronic pain. The object of 'needle surgery' in treating unstable joints is to inject a sclerosing agent into the ligaments, causing the contraction and thickening of the ligament, thus strengthening its supporting effect on that joint." Boyd is describing Prolotherapy. [9]

Boyd continues by saying that the cause of back pain in a so-called ruptured disc is not pressure of the disc on nerve roots, as orthopedic surgeons would have you believe, because the disc is absorbed by the body in a few weeks. The back hurts in such cases because once the disc has disappeared, the spinal column loses vertical height and the ligaments become too long and loose to keep the structure stable. This instability and unwanted motion create core irritation, congestion, and inflammation. [10]

Surgery and other invasive treatments are directed at relieving pain but not relieving the underlying condition that caused the pain in the first place. What happens when you cover up a problem and do not solve it? Can you imagine "solving" your financial problems by paying your bills with your credit card? By doing so, your financial problems actually worsen. When treatments cover up the pain without correcting the underlying problem, the initial condition that caused the pain may actually worsen. The person may require more and more pain medicine or other treatments in order to alleviate the pain. It is our hope that by educating more patients and physicians about Prolotherapy we can end the onslaught of these procedures and correct the "true" underlying cause of the pain. ■

CHAPTER 3

Why Prolotherapy Works

"A joint is only as strong as its weakest ligament."
—George S. Hackett, M.D.

Simply put, pain is due to weakness. If our buddy Joe and Ross were to pick up a piano, we can guarantee they wouldn't be holding it long. After a few seconds, Joe's back would be hurting and about everything on Ross would be aching. We would be in pain because, unlike Hercules, we are too weak to lift a piano. Likewise, most neck, back, and other musculoskeletal pains are due to weakness, specifically weakness in the ligaments and tendons.

"Ligament relaxation is a condition in which the strength of the ligament fibers has become impaired so that a stretching of the fibrous strands occurs when the ligament is submitted to normal or less than normal tension."[1] This statement was made 40 years ago by George S. Hackett, M.D., who believed chronic pain was simply due to ligament weakness in and around the joint. Dr. Hackett coined the phrase "ligament and tendon relaxation" which is synonymous with ligament and tendon weakness, and subsequently developed the treatment known as Prolotherapy.

PROLOTHERAPY DEFINED

Webster's Third New International Dictionary defines Prolotherapy as "the rehabilitation of an incompetent structure, such as a ligament or tendon, by the induced proliferation of new cells."[2] Prolotherapy is the injection of substances at the site where ligaments and tendons attach to the bone, thus stimulating the ligaments and tendons to proliferate or grow at the injection site. This area is called the fibro-osseous junction. "Fibro" means fibrous tissue which forms the ligament or tendon, and "osseous" refers to the bone.

Prolotherapy works because it addresses and corrects the root cause of chronic pain: ligament and tendon relaxation.

LIGAMENTS AND TENDONS

A strain is defined as a stretched or injured tendon. A sprain is a stretched or injured ligament. Blood flow is vital to the body's healing process and, because ligaments and tendons have naturally poor blood supply, incomplete healing may result after an injury to that structure.[3, 4] This incomplete healing results in decreased strength of the area. The ligaments and tendons, normally taut and thus strong bands of fibrous or connective tissue, become relaxed and weak. The weakened ligament or tendon then becomes the source of the chronic pain.

Ligaments and tendons are bands of tissue consisting of various amino acids in a matrix called collagen. Tendons attach the muscles to the surface of the bone, enabling movement of the joints and bones. Ligaments attach one bone to another, thus preventing overextension of bones and joints. **(See Figure 3-1.)**

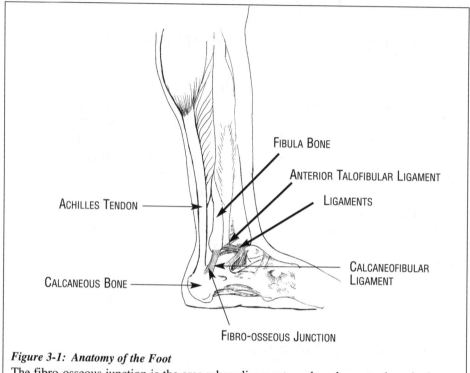

FIBULA BONE

ANTERIOR TALOFIBULAR LIGAMENT

LIGAMENTS

ACHILLES TENDON

CALCANEOFIBULAR LIGAMENT

CALCANEOUS BONE

FIBRO-OSSEOUS JUNCTION

Figure 3-1: Anatomy of the Foot
The fibro-osseous junction is the area where ligaments and tendons attach to the bone.

Damage to ligaments and tendons will cause excessive movement of the joints resulting in chronic pain. Damage to ligaments causes joints to become loose or weak and often manifests itself with a cracking sensation during movement. Tendon weakness produces painful and weak joints.

For example, there are many causes of chronic elbow pain including the tennis elbow (extensor tendonitis), annular ligament sprain, and biceps muscle strain. Since muscle, ligament, or tendon injury can all cause pain, a proper diagnosis is needed to permanently alleviate the pain. Tennis elbow is diagnosed when the physician notices weakness and pain with wrist extension and tenderness at the elbow where the extensor tendons attach. Annular ligament sprain is diagnosed by the physician palpating this ligament in the elbow and eliciting a positive "jump sign." **(See Figure 3-2.)**

Another source of elbow pain is biceps muscle strain. When the biceps tendon is weak, resisted flexion (resisting the upward movement of the forearm) of the elbow is painful. Since the bicep muscle flexes at the elbow, carrying a box or turning a screwdriver may produce the painful symptoms associated with strain or weakness of this muscle. Since the extensor tendons, bicep muscle, and annular lig-

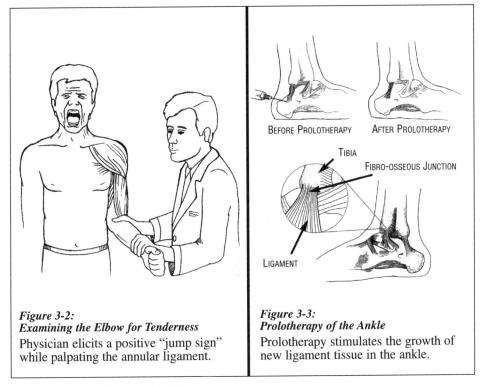

Figure 3-2:
Examining the Elbow for Tenderness
Physician elicits a positive "jump sign" while palpating the annular ligament.

Figure 3-3:
Prolotherapy of the Ankle
Prolotherapy stimulates the growth of new ligament tissue in the ankle.

ament all attach to the bone in the elbow, good palpatory skills are necessary for proper diagnosis. Prolotherapy is given at the fibro-osseous junction where the positive "jump sign" is elicited. Prolotherapy causes proliferation, or growth of tissue at this point. **(See Figure 3-3.)** Prolotherapy will strengthen the muscle, tendon, or ligament tissue at the fibro-osseous junction which is needed to alleviate pain.

WHAT ARE LIGAMENTS AND TENDONS?

The most sensitive structures that produce pain according to Daniel Kayfetz, M.D., are the periosteum and the ligaments. It is important to note that in the scale of pain sensitivity (which part of the body hurts more when injured), Dr. Kayfetz notes that the periosteum (outer layer of bone) ranks first, followed by ligaments, tendons, fascia (the connective tissue that surrounds muscle), and finally muscle. Articular (joint) cartilage contains no sensory nerve endings. The area where the ligaments attach to the bone is the fibro-osseous junction. This is why injury to this area is so significant. It causes massive amounts of pain. This is where the Prolotherapy injections occur and thus the strengthening of these areas and subsequent relief of pain.[5]

Ligaments provide stability of the joints. If joints move too much, the bones may compress or pinch nerves or blood vessels resulting in permanent nerve damage. Weakened structures are strengthened by the growth of new, strong ligament and tendon tissue induced by the Prolotherapy injections. This is illustrated in a relatively common back condition called spondylolisthesis. A weak area of bone, in conjunction with stretched ligaments, allow vertebrae to slip and pinch a nerve, resulting in terrible back pain and radiating pain down the leg. Prolotherapy strengthens the weakened areas and realigns the vertebrae, relieving the pinched nerve and eliminating the chronic pain. **(See Figures 3-4.)**

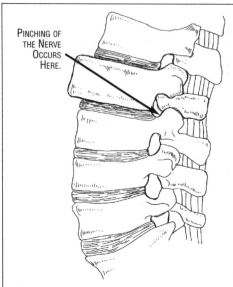

PINCHING OF THE NERVE OCCURS HERE.

Figure 3-4A:
Spondylolisthesis—Slippage of the Vertebrae
Weakened ligaments lead to spondylolis-
thesis and pinching of the nerves.

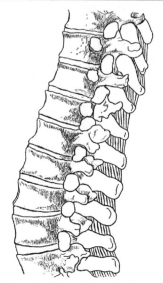

Figure 3-4B: Proper Vertebral Alignment
After Prolotherapy
Prolotherapy strengthens the ligaments
and joints that support the vertebrae to
move into proper alignment and relieves
nerve pinching.

THE ROLE OF PROLOTHERAPY

Prolotherapy permanently strengthens tissue. Strengthening weakened structures produces permanent pain relief. Prolotherapy effectively eliminates pain
because it attacks the source of the pain: the fibro-osseous junction, an area rich
in sensory nerves.[6,7] When a weakened ligament or tendon is stretched, the sensory nerves become irritated, causing local and referred pain throughout the body.
These referred pain patterns of ligaments were outlined in Dr. Hackett's observations after he performed more than 18,000 intraligamentous injections to 1,656
patients over a period of 19 years.[8]

A referred pain occurs when a local ligament injury sends pain to another area
of the body. Dr. Hackett described the referral patterns of the ligaments involving
the hip, pelvis, lower back, and neck. **(See Figures 2-2, 3, 4.)** Physical therapists,
chiropractors, family physicians, and orthopedists are usually unaware of liga-

ment referral pain patterns. From the illustration, note that the hip ligaments refer pain to the big toe. The sacroiliac ligaments refer pain to the lateral foot, which causes the symptoms resulting in a common misdiagnosis of "sciatica." Pain traveling down the back into the leg and foot is usually from ligament weakness in the sacroiliac joint, not pinching of the sciatic nerve. Patients who are misdiagnosed with "sciatica" are often subjected to numerous tests, anti-inflammatory medicines, and surgical procedures with unsatisfactory results. Prolotherapy eliminates the local ligament pain, as well as the referred pain, and is curative in most cases of sciatica.

Ligament injuries may cause crushing severe pain because the ligaments are full of nerves, some of the nerve tissue being free nerve endings.[9, 10] Movement may aggravate the damaged nerve in the ligament and produces a shock-like sensation, giving the impression that a nerve is being pinched. It is a nerve-type pain that is due to a ligament stretching, not a nerve pinching. When a weak ligament is stretched, the nerves inside the ligament often send shock-like pain to distant sites, as in sciatica pain. If the ligament is strengthened with Prolotherapy, the nerves in the ligaments do not fire, thereby relieving the pain.

It is well-known that an injury in one segment of the body can affect other distant body parts, especially in regard to ligament injury. For example, when dye is injected into the nerves of the ligaments of the lower neck, the dye will travel four segments above and four segments below the initial injection site. The dye may be seen in the autonomic (sympathetic) nerves in these areas.[11] This implies that ligament laxity at one vertebral level could manifest pain, muscle tension, adrenal, or automatic dysfunction four segments above or below the actual injury site. This is one of the explanations as to why ligament pain is often diffuse and can take on a burning quality.

Knowledge of referral pain patterns, along with a complete patient medical history, allows physicians who practice Prolotherapy to make accurate diagnoses of specific weak ligaments, even before performing an examination. A Prolotherapist, for example, may examine a back pain patient with pain radiating down the leg to the knee. This reveals that the source of the pain is likely the "A" and "B" areas of the sacroiliac ligaments. (**As seen in Figures 2-3 and 2-4.**) Pain continuing to the lateral foot indicates weak "D" area sacroiliac ligaments. Pain radiating to the big toe reveals the source is in the hip area.

The physician examines the appropriate area utilizing his most important diagnostic tool—the thumb. We call it our personal MRI scanner: My Reproducibility Instrument. A diagnosis is made when a positive "jump sign" is observed. This occurs when the injured ligament is palpated, causing the patient to jump off the examination table due to the severe tenderness of the ligament. The pain is caused by something between the pressing thumb and the bone. The something between these two areas is the ligament. (**See Figure 3-5.**) The positive "jump sign" gives both patient and physician confidence that the pain-producing structure has been

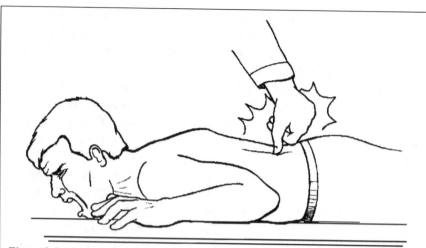

Figure 3-5
Physician Eliciting a Positive "Jump Sign"
The best MRI scanner is **M**y **R**eproducibility **I**nstrument—which is the thumb.

identified. Ligament injuries are often not detected with CAT or MRI scans because ligaments are such small structures. If a positive "jump sign" can be elicited, then permanent pain relief with Prolotherapy is likely.

Prolotherapy is so successful because it attacks the root cause of chronic pain which is most commonly ligament laxity (weakness). Signs of ligament laxity or injury are the following: **1.** chronic pain, **2.** referral pain patterns, **3.** tender areas, **4.** positive "jump signs," **5.** pain aggravated by movement, **6.** cracking sensation in the joint when moved, **7.** chronic subluxation, or **8.** temporary help from physical therapy, massage, or chiropractic manipulation. Prolotherapy helps strengthen chronically weak ligaments and relieves all of the above.

In summary, Prolotherapy works by permanently strengthening the ligament, muscle, and tendon attachments to the bone, the fibro-osseous junction. Because the cause of pain is addressed, Prolotherapy is often curative. ■

CHAPTER 4

Prolotherapy Provides Results

Prolotherapy is effective because it attacks and eliminates the root cause of chronic pain: ligament and tendon relaxation. Ligament relaxation causes joints to loosen. A weak ligament will have difficulty holding a joint in place. The nerve fibers within the weakened ligament are activated and cause local pain. They may also cause a referred pain pattern as shown in **Figure 2-4.** The muscles surrounding the loose ligament contract to help stabilize the joint—the reason why people with loose ligaments and chronic pain have tight, painful muscles. Only when the weakened ligaments are strengthened will the local and referred pain patterns, as well as the muscle pain, subside. The same is true for tendon weakness.

Research has been conducted exhibiting the effectiveness of Prolotherapy. The following studies are just a sample of the research that has been done during the past 40 years.

GEORGE S. HACKETT, M.D.

Although chronic pain has many causes, the vast majority of chronic pain sufferers have loose joints caused by ligament weakness. This is evidenced by George S. Hackett, M.D.'s research study described in the third edition of his book, *Ligament and Tendon Relaxation Treated by Prolotherapy*, published in 1958.[1] The study consisted of the following:

- sample size: 656 patients
- patient age range: 15 to 88 years old
- duration of pain prior to treatment: three months to 65 years
- average duration of pain prior to treatment: four-and-a-half years
- duration of study: 19 years
- number of injections given: 18,000

Twelve years after the Prolotherapy treatment was completed, 82 percent of the patients considered themselves cured. Dr. Hackett believed that the cure rate with Prolotherapy was over 90 percent due to improvements in the technique over the years.

In 1955, Dr. Hackett analyzed 146 consecutive cases of undiagnosed low back disability during a two-month period. He found that 94 percent of the patients experienced joint ligament relaxation. In 1956, a similar survey of 124 consecutive cases of undiagnosed low back disability revealed that 97 percent of patients possessed joint instability from ligament weakness. The sacroiliac ligaments were involved in 75 percent of the low back ligament laxity cases. The lumbosacral ligaments were involved in 54 percent. He also noted that approximately 50 percent had already undergone back surgery for a previous diagnosis of a disc problem.[2]

At this time, Prolotherapy produced an 80 percent cure rate even though 50 percent of the people treated had undergone back surgery. Obviously, the surgical procedures did not relieve the patients' back pain. Rarely does a disc problem cause disabling back pain. Chronic pain in the lower back is most commonly due to ligament weakness—the reason Prolotherapy is so effective.

Dr. Hackett attributed ineffective response to Prolotherapy to: **1.** inability to clearly confirm the diagnosis by the injection of a local anesthetic solution, **2.** failure of the patient to return for completion of the treatment, **3.** treatment in the presence of another disability, **4.** a less refined technique and less experience in the earlier studies, **5.** lowered morale from years of suffering and disappointment from unsuccessful treatments and dependence on prescription pain medications, and **6.** non-responsiveness to the stimulation of proliferation.

Prolotherapy works because it causes ligament and tendon growth. Dr. Hackett used Sylnasol, a sodium salt fatty acid, as a proliferant in his original work. Animals were given between one and three injections of the proliferating solution into the tendon and the fibro-osseous junction. There was no necrosis (dead tissue) noted in any of the specimens. No destruction of nerves, blood vessels, or tendinous bands was noted. Compared to non-injected tendons, tendons treated with Prolotherapy showed a 40 percent increase in diameter. The fibro-osseous junction, where the tendon attaches to bone, increased by 30 percent, forming permanent tendon tissue. Dr. Hackett believed the 40 percent increase in diameter of the tendon represented a doubling of the tendon strength.[3]

GUSTAV A. HEMWALL, M.D.

Gustav A. Hemwall, M.D., learned the technique of Prolotherapy from Dr. Hackett and then proceeded to treat more than 10,000 patients worldwide. He collected data on 8,000 of those patients. In 1974, Dr. Hemwall presented his largest survey of 2,007 Prolotherapy patients to the Prolotherapy Association. The survey related the following:

- 1,871 patients completed treatment
- 6,000 Prolotherapy treatments were administered
- 1,399 (75.5 percent) patients reported complete recovery and cure
- 413 (24.3 percent) reported general improvement
- 25 (0.2 percent) patients showed no improvement
- 170 patients were lost to follow-up

More than 99 percent of the patients who completed treatment with Prolotherapy found relief from their chronic pain. These results are similar to those published by Dr. Hackett, showing that Prolotherapy is completely curative in many cases and provides some pain relief in nearly all.[4]

Y. KING LIU, PH.D.

In 1983, Y. King Liu performed a study using the knee ligament in rabbits.[5] This study was done to confirm Dr. Hackett's earlier work and better quantify the strength of the tissue formed by Prolotherapy. In this study, a five percent sodium morrhuate solution, an extract of cod liver oil, was injected into the femoral and tibial attachments of the medial collateral ligament, the inside knee ligament.

The ligaments were injected five times and then compared to non-injected ligaments. The results showed that in every case Prolotherapy significantly increased ligamentous mass, thickness, and cross-sectional area as well as the ligament strength. In a six-week period, ligament mass increased by 44 percent, ligament thickness by 27 percent, and the ligament-bone junction strength by 28 percent. This research was yet another attestation to the effectiveness of Prolotherapy, showing that Prolotherapy actually causes new tissue to grow.

THE EFFECTS OF FIVE PROLOTHERAPY TREATMENTS TO THE MEDIAL COLLATERAL LIGAMENT

	Prolotherapy-Injected Ligaments	Saline-Injected Ligaments (Control)	% Change
Ligament Mass (mg)	132.2	89.7	44
Ligament Thickness (mm)	1.01	0.79	27
Ligament Mass Length (mg/mm)	6.45	4.39	47
Junction Strength (N)	119.1	93.5	28

Figure 4-1: The Effects of Five Prolotherapy Treatments to the Medial Collateral Ligament Prolotherapy causes a statistically significant increase in ligament mass and strength as well as bone-ligament junction strength.

J. A. MAYNARD, M.D.

To confirm the work of Dr. Liu and describe how the proliferants in Prolotherapy grow tissue, J.A. Maynard, M.D., and associates, treated rabbit tendons with proliferant solutions. After the proliferant injections, the actual tendon circumferences increased an average of 20 to 25 percent after six weeks.

They found that "the increase in circumference appeared to be due to an increase in cell population [immune cells], water content, and ground substance [glue that holds the collagen together].... Consequently, not only is there an increase in the number of cells but also a wider variety of cell types, fibroblasts, neutrophils, lymphocytes, plasma cells, and unidentifiable cells in the injected tissues."[6]

The findings were similar to what normally occurs when injured tissue is repairing itself. Prolotherapy induces the normal healing mechanisms of the body.

After Prolotherapy, there is increased circulation bringing with it not only nutrients, but cells. These immune cells then begin the growth of collagen tissue to rebuild the injured tissue. Eventually, new collagen tissue forms, creating stronger ligaments and tendons.[7]

ROBERT KLEIN, M.D.

In human studies, Robert Klein, M.D., and associates, administered a series of six weekly injections in the lower back ligamentous supporting structures with a proliferant solution containing Dextrose, glycerin, and phenol. Biopsies performed three months after completion of injections showed statistically significant increases in collagen fiber and ligament diameter by 60 percent. Statistically significant improvements in pain relief and back motion were also observed.[8]

THOMAS DORMAN, M.D.

In a 1989 study, Thomas Dorman, M.D., noted, "I biopsied individuals before and after treatment with Prolotherapy and submitted the biopsy specimens to pathologists. Using modern analytic techniques, they showed that Prolotherapy caused regrowth of tissue, an increased number of fibroblast nuclei, (the major cell type in ligaments and other connective tissue), an increased amount of collagen, and an absence of inflammatory changes or other types of tissue damage."[9]

Dr. Dorman performed a retrospective survey of 80 patients treated with Prolotherapy for cervical, thoracic, lumbar spine pain, or a combination of these. Thirty-one percent of the patients had litigation or workman's compensation cases. The patients were evaluated up to five years after their Prolotherapy treatment. Analysis of the 80 patients showed a statistical significance of $P<.001$ for improvements in **1.** severity of pain, **2.** daily living activities, and **3.** influence of sleep pattern. Prolotherapy was shown to eliminate pain, improve activity level, and help the patients get a good night's sleep.[10]

MILNE ONGLEY, M.D.

Using the same solution as Dr. Klein, Milne Ongley, M.D., and associates, demonstrated a stabilization of the collateral and cruciate ligaments of the knee joint with Prolotherapy. All subjects treated showed an increase in activity and reduction in pain.[11] Two double-blind studies where patients received either a proliferant injected solution or a solution without proliferant concluded that Prolotherapy was effective in eliminating pain.[12, 13]

A problem with controlled studies using Prolotherapy injections is that the control group still receives an injection, though without any proliferant. An injection into a tender area is a treatment utilized in pain management. The result is that the control group actually receives a therapeutic intervention. Despite these concerns, Prolotherapy in the above two studies was shown to be an effective treatment for chronic low back pain.

ROBERT SCHWARTZ, M.D.

In another study, by Robert Schwartz, M.D., on the effects of Prolotherapy on 43 patients with chronic low back pain who had been unresponsive to other treatments including surgery, Prolotherapy treatments were given over a six-week period into and around the sacroiliac joint. At two weeks, 20 of 43 patients reported 95 percent improvement, 31 of 43 patients reported 75 percent or better improvement, and 35 of 43 reported 66 percent or better improvement. Only three of 43 reported no improvement. The result of this study of chronic resistant low back pain, revealed that 93 percent of the patients experienced pain relief with Prolotherapy after the six weeks.[14]

HAROLD WILKINSON, M.D.

Between 1979 and 1995, Harold Wilkinson, M.D., a professor and former chairman of the Division of Neurosurgery at the University of Massachusetts Medical Center who has been practicing Prolotherapy for 30 years, gave 349 posterior iliac Prolotherapy injections for chronic low back pain. Generally, the patients had undergone prior spinal operations and had been referred to him because they were "failed back patients." In other words, no one could help them. Of the 349 injections, one injection totally relieved 29 percent of the patients, and a total of 76 percent of the patients received significant pain relief with one injection. A full 93 percent of the people received pain relief with only one Prolotherapy injection in the lower back.[15]

In regard to other areas of the body besides the lower back, Dr. Wilkinson reported on results of 115 Prolotherapy injections. Forty-three percent of these completely eliminated the person's pain and 89 percent of the patients, with only one Prolotherapy injection, received some pain relief. Dr. Wilkinson, in compiling the data, stated that it was noteworthy that "a sizeable portion of people with unresolved chronic pain had more than a year's pain relief with only one Prolotherapy injection."

Dr. Wilkinson explained that exercise and massage help trigger points (tender points) originating from muscles by increasing blood circulation but these treatments do not help ligamentous or periosteal (fibro-osseous) trigger points. This is because just increasing blood circulation is not enough to grow the new ligament tissue. Prolotherapy must be done to stimulate the growth of ligamentous tissue at the periosteal junction.

CONFIRMING DIAGNOSIS

There are two aspects by which the correct diagnosis can be completely and reliably confirmed without extensive tests. The first method involves palpating the area involved until a positive "jump sign" is elicited. If a patient's pain can be reproduced by manual palpation, the prognosis for complete relief with Prolotherapy is excellent.

The second method of confirming the diagnosis is by the Prolotherapy treatment itself. The Prolotherapy solution contains various proliferants along with an anesthetic. Prolotherapy is one of the few treatments that actually treats the condition while confirming the diagnosis. Since Prolotherapy injections are given where the ligaments and tendons attach to the bone (fibro-osseous junction) the patient will feel immediate pain relief after the treatment, if the diagnosis is correct. This is due to the effect of the local anesthetic blocking the pain coming from the injured ligaments and tendons. Immediate pain relief after Prolotherapy treatments, along with the reproducibility of the pain when the ligament or tendon is palpated, gives both the patient and the physician confidence that the diagnosis of ligament and tendon relaxation is correct.

SUMMARY

Prolotherapy works because an accurate diagnosis of ligament and tendon weakness can be confirmed by an appropriate patient history and a reproduction of the pain by direct palpation of the injured structure. The pain is immediately alleviated due to the effect of the anesthetic from the Prolotherapy solution. This provides further confirmation that the diagnosis of ligament and tendon relaxation is correct.

Prolotherapy causes a thickening of ligament and tendon tissue. This increases the strength of the ligament and tendon and causes the chronic pain to subside. According to Dr. Hackett and Dr. Hemwall, Prolotherapy is more than 90 percent effective in either eliminating chronic pain or significantly decreasing pain complaints. It is for these reasons that many people are choosing to Prolo their chronic pain away. ■

CHAPTER 5

Answers to Common Questions about Prolotherapy

A fter years of suffering from chronic pain, many people find it hard to believe that there is a treatment they haven't heard about, that it has the potential to cure them, and on top of it, has been around for 50 years. As hard as it is to believe, there is a treatment that can cure chronic pain and yes, Prolotherapy has been around for 50 years.

We enjoy questions. Ross once asked Marion if she thought he was the greatest. She replied, "You're the greatest person I know to get us into a fiasco." That was not the answer he was looking for! Anyone contemplating any procedure, including Prolotherapy, should have all of their questions answered. They should also understand why they are getting the procedure and what it is supposed to accomplish.

1. DO PROLOTHERAPY INJECTIONS HURT?

As the saying goes with body builders, it also goes with Prolotherapy, "no pain, no gain." Shots are shots. "Do they hurt?" every new patient asks, as sweat begins to form on the patient's forehead and palms as the needle approaches its target. Let us put it to you this way—our patients begin to sweat when they see us in the grocery store. We don't know why, we're nice people! All doctors were taught the appropriate answer to this question in medical school. "It hurts a little." Does anything the doctor sticks you with really hurt just a little? Some people have many Prolotherapy injections and do not flinch, while others receive a few shots and have a rough time.

A good friend and an expert in Orthopedic Medicine, Rodney Van Pelt, M.D., told us the following story about his first Prolotherapy experience. He once attended a conference where Gustav A. Hemwall, M.D., the world's most experienced Prolotherapist, discussed the technique and asked for a volunteer to help illustrate an actual Prolotherapy procedure. So, Dr. Van Pelt, being the adventuresome Californian that he is, jumped out of his seat and volunteered.

For many years, Dr. Van Pelt had suffered from back pain without finding a curative treatment. Due to the deteriorated state of his back, he required quite a number of Prolotherapy injections. Before Dr. Hemwall had finished the treatment, the pain from the injections caused Dr. Van Pelt to pass out. Dr. Hemwall just went on injecting and instructing the physicians on the use of Prolotherapy for chronic low back pain. He then informed the audience that he would rather treat 100 women than one man.

Let's face it. God made women to be able to deliver babies. It has been said that if men were to deliver babies, the human race would become extinct. The amount of pain experienced during the Prolotherapy treatment is insignificant compared to the pain the chronic pain patient experiences every day. Many say after the Prolotherapy treatment, "It wasn't that bad." There are a few people, however, like Dr. Van Pelt, who need a little pampering.

Pampering to lessen the pain may consist of the physician giving the patient anesthesia or a prescription for Tylenol with codeine or Vicodin to be taken prior to Prolotherapy treatments. Other physicians, including Dr. Hemwall and Dr. Hauser, use a device called Madajet which sprays an anesthetic such as Lidocaine into the skin to deaden the pain when the needle pierces the skin. The needle piercing through the skin is the most painful part of the procedure.

For those requiring injections in many areas at one time or in very delicate areas like the neck, intravenous anesthesia such as Demerol, which is a narcotic, may be used. The intravenous anesthesia is the most dangerous part of the procedure. An occasional nausea and a few "upchucks" were the only side effects Dr. Hemwall witnessed after administering thousands of intravenous anesthetics. The anesthesia does make a person "woozy" but some people prefer it because it eliminates the pain of the procedure. Most of our patients receive Prolotherapy without any anesthesia and do quite well.

2. How Safe Is Prolotherapy?

In his study published in 1961, Abraham Myers, M.D., states that in treating 267 patients with low back pain with and without sciatica from May 1956 to October 1960 "over 4,500 [Prolotherapy] injections have been given without the occurrence of any complication."[1]

Prolotherapy is much safer than taking aspirin day after day. Prolotherapy is also much safer for the body than living with pain. The most dangerous part of receiving Prolotherapy treatments at our office is fighting Chicago traffic!

Pain not only decreases one's enjoyment of life, it creates stress in the body. Stress is the worst detriment to good health. A body under stress triggers the "fight or flight" response, which means the adrenal gland begins excreting hormones such as cortisol and adrenaline. The same thing occurs when a gun is pointed at you during a robbery, but for a shorter period of time.

The adrenal gland, also known as the stress gland, secretes cortisol to increase the amount of white blood cells that are activated, as in cases of allergic or infectious stress. It puts the body "on alert." The adrenal gland is one of the reasons a person wakes up in the morning. Chronic pain causes the adrenal gland to be in a continual "alert mode," secreting cortisol as would occur with an infection, or when a person is being robbed. As the chronic pain lingers, cortisol is continually produced. Cortisol levels are supposed to be low at night time, putting the body in the sleep mode. With chronic pain, high cortisol levels put the body in the alert mode and insomnia results. The increased cortisol production eventually wears the body down, resulting in increased fatigue. This explains why many chronic pain patients have difficulty sleeping and complain of non-restful sleep.

The adrenal gland also secretes adrenaline, more properly named epinephrine, which is the hormone that stimulates the sympathetic nervous system. When the sympathetic nervous system is activated, blood vessels constrict and blood pressure rises—an unhealthy situation long-term. This produces free radicals, causing oxidative damage to the body. Long-term stress from chronic pain results in long-term oxidative damage. This is one reason that people who suffer from chronic pain are ill more frequently and age prematurely. This can also explain why they seem "stressed out." Physiologically, they are! For chronic pain patients, the only way to turn off the adrenaline system is to eliminate the pain. If the chronic pain is due to ligament or tendon laxity, Prolotherapy is required.

Pain causes enormous stress on the body which further enhances the need to rid the body of the pain. Prolotherapy is recommended for every patient with structural chronic pain. Structural pain from a loose joint, cartilage, muscle, tendon, or ligament weakness can be eliminated with Prolotherapy.

Dr. Hemwall, who treated more than 10,000 patients with more than four million injections, had not one episode of paralysis, death, permanent nerve injury, or infection. In the words of Dr. Hemwall, "not even a pimple" has formed at the site of the injections. It is common, however, to experience muscle stiffness after the injections for a few days.

3. WHAT ABOUT PRESCRIPTION NARCOTICS?

Dr. Hemwall prescribed analgesics like Tylenol with codeine to ease stiffness and pain after Prolotherapy treatments. We occasionally use codeine, but we more commonly use Tylenol, Ultram (which do not decrease inflammation), or natural analgesics like bromelain or natural muscle relaxers such as magnesium. We **do not** recommend chronic use of narcotic medications like codeine, Vicodin, or Darvocet. These are wonderful pain killers, but chronic pain is never due to a Tylenol with codeine deficiency. Chronic pain always has a cause. If that cause is eliminated, the pain will disappear.

Most people understand the addictive quality of narcotics. This is a good reason not to use narcotics for more than a few days. Another reason to avoid narcotics is that narcotic medications suppress the immune system.

Chronic use of narcotics has been shown to decrease both B-cell and T-cell function, reduce the effectiveness of phagocytes to kill organisms like Candida and cause atrophy of such important immune organs as the spleen and thymus.[2,3] The spleen and thymus glands are two structures in the body that are vital to helping the immune system fight off infections. Another study on the use of narcotics concluded that people with the potential for bacterial or viral infections should be cautioned against the use of narcotic medication.[4]

Narcotic medications, because of their potential immune-suppressing effect as well as their addictive properties, should be used as little as possible. Narcotic medications, as indicated above, can cause the shrinking of such important glands as the thymus and spleen.

A much more viable option than suppressing the pain with narcotic medications is to determine the root cause of the pain and correct it. Prolotherapy accomplishes this. If pain medicine is needed, Tylenol or Ultram can be used because they do not suppress inflammation. Anti-inflammatory medications, such as Motrin, Advil, or Voltaren, cannot be used because they suppress inflammation and block the beneficial effects of the Prolotherapy. Most people with chronic pain admit that they want to stop using pain medications. Often they say, "I just don't feel right being on those." Of course not. Would you feel "right" if your spleen and thymus were shrinking?

4. How Many Treatments are Necessary and How Often?

The anesthetic in the solution used during Prolotherapy sessions often provides immediate pain relief. The pain relief may continue after the effect of the anesthetic subsides due to the stabilizing of the treated joints because of the inflammation caused by the Prolotherapy injections. This pain relief normally continues for a few weeks after the first treatment.

Between the second and fourth weeks, the initial stabilization induced by the Prolotherapy subsides, and because the initial growth of ligament tissue is not complete, some of the original pain may return during this "window period" of healing. Follow-up is recommended six weeks after each treatment to ensure an accurate assessment of results, avoiding an evaluation of a patient during the "window period." Prolotherapy is performed every six weeks because most ligaments heal over a six-week period.[5] **(See Figure 5-1.)**

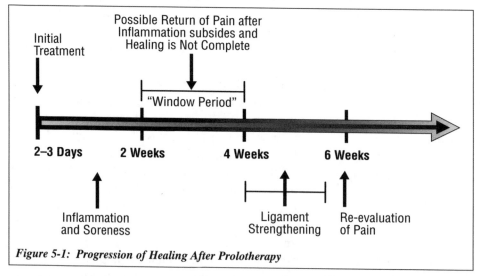

Figure 5-1: Progression of Healing After Prolotherapy

As healing progresses, the quantity of injections required per treatment usually decreases. The pain generally continues to diminish with each treatment until it is completely eliminated. Four to six treatments are normally required to eliminate pain. Because everyone is unique, some people may only require one treatment while others will require as many as eight treatments. Rarely are more needed.

In some cases, patients will experience no pain relief after their first or second Prolotherapy treatments. This does not mean the therapy is not working, rather it is an indication that the ligaments and tendons are not yet strong enough to stabilize the joints. The amount of collagen growth required for stabilization of the joint is different for each person. A patient who experiences pain relief at rest but not during activity requires further treatment to strengthen the area. If Prolotherapy treatments are continued, there is an excellent chance of achieving total pain relief with the resumption of all previous activities.

All prospective patients who receive disability insurance or workman's compensation, are involved in a legal matter, or are on a leave of absence from work, are told that the ultimate goal of Prolotherapy treatments is to help them return to normal function, including returning to work. In individuals who do not have a real desire to return to work or discontinue receiving disability insurance, Prolotherapy is not indicated. In such cases, the individuals do not possess a "real" desire to heal and Prolotherapy will not ease the pain, as pain relief would be an admission that disability checks are no longer needed.

The above situation is a rarity in our office. The overwhelming majority of people suffering from chronic pain desire to find pain relief and return to work. A few patients have a phobia of needles. For those individuals, other Natural Medicine treatments are prescribed, but the results are significantly less dramatic than what is expected with Prolotherapy. Herbs and vitamins will not stabilize a chronically loose joint. Exercise will not stabilize a chronically loose joint. Prolotherapy is the one treatment that will. There is no substitute for Prolotherapy with regard to curing pain.

Patients who do not attain pain relief because of a phobia of needles, or give up on Prolotherapy after one or two sessions because of slower than expected pain relief are needlessly living with chronic pain, especially when a conservative, curative treatment is available. The number one reason for partial pain relief with Prolotherapy is not completing the full course of Prolotherapy sessions. It is important that the patient does not become disappointed if the pain is not relieved after one or two sessions, especially a patient who has been in pain for decades. We have seen severe pain cases require only one treatment and relatively simple cases require six sessions.

Overcoming phobias and fears is difficult but worthwhile, and it often produces the most happiness. Ross's phobia was girls. In high school, he was often too scared to ask a girl for a date. There was one particular girl's picture he fell in love with when he was 12 years of age while looking through his year book at Jack Benny Junior High School in Waukegan, Illinois. It wasn't until after high school graduation that he was brave enough to call her. We talked and laughed for hours at Bevier Park in Waukegan, Illinois, on July 19, 1980. Twenty years later, we are still talking and laughing. We're sure glad that he had the courage to call Marion that day. Our lives would be pretty empty without each other! We must often overcome our fears to enjoy the true happiness that life offers.

5. IS PROLOTHERAPY COVERED BY INSURANCE?

Some insurance companies cover Prolotherapy while others do not. The usual reason for denying coverage is that Prolotherapy is not a "usual and customary treatment." **(See Figure 5-2.)**

ThePrudential

Jan Behm
Claim Consultant
Illinois Group Claim Division

The Prudential Insurance Company of America
P.O. Box 567
Matteson, IL 60443-0567
(708) 503-7360

April 2, 1993

G.A. Hemwall, M.D.
715 Lake St.
Oak Park, IL 60302

Re:
SS#:

Dear Dr. Hemwall:

We have completed our review of   claim file as it pertains to the prolotherapy rendered to her on 4/11/92, 5/30/92 & 8/15/92.

Her claim file, along with the additional information you submitted, has been reviewed by our local Medical Department and our Corporate Office. As a result, we find that prolotherapy or proliferant therapy is considered an acceptable form of treatment for pain relief and for breaking down calcification around ligaments. Accordingly, benefits will be released for the services rendered 5/30/92 & 8/15/92. (Payment was already made for the treatment on 4/11/92.)

Please accept our apologies for the delay in replying to your last appeal. Should you have any questions, please feel free to contact our office.

Sincerely,

Jan Behm
Claim Consultant
Illinois Group Claim Division

JB:dr

Figure 5-2: Typical Letter Approving Insurance Reimbursement for Prolotherapy
Patients must educate insurance companies about Prolotherapy in order to obtain reimbursements

---

The Chicago Medical Society, a branch of the American Medical Association (AMA), reviewed a case for Aetna Life & Casualty Company and submitted the following on April 20, 1976 to Dr. Hemwall regarding their decision: "In response to the insurance carrier's request of whether your treatment [Prolotherapy] is an approved and appropriate method, the Subcommittee on Insurance Mediation has made a decision on the above entitled matter. On the basis of the information presented, it is the Committee's opinion that this procedure is an accepted procedure." [6] **(See Appendix F, Insurance Reimbursement Letters.)**

A few years later, the procedure was again reviewed by the Chicago Medical Society. In a letter dated November 1, 1979 to the Life Investors Insurance Company of America, the chairman of the Medical Practice Committee wrote, "It is the opinion of the Committee that, while the treatment does not enjoy widespread acceptance in medical circles, it is a well recognized procedure in veterinary medicine: animal models of disease and treatment form the basis for a great deal of medical knowledge and progress. It is significant to this Committee that Dr. Hemwall has performed this procedure on a great many people over an eighteen year period of time and our Society has never received a patient complaint on the procedure. It appears to us that this record speaks for successful treatment. We do not feel that either we, or an insurance carrier, are in a position to declare an uncommon, but apparently successful, procedure as an improper one. Because the method is not widely used does not mean that it is not compensable. A search of our records reveals that another Committee of our Society was presented with a similar question regarding 'Prolotherapy' (the previous reference) and they found it an accepted procedure and recommended payment of the physicians fees. We agree." [7]

The third time the Chicago Medical Society reviewed Prolotherapy was on November 5, 1987. Peter C. Pulos, M.D., Chairman of the Medical Practice Committee wrote this concerning Prolotherapy, "We understand that this procedure has been used by many medical and osteopathic physicians both in this country and in Europe. It is significant that Dr. Hemwall has performed this procedure on many people for almost 30 years and our Society has never received a complaint on the use of the procedure. It appears to the committee that this record speaks for successful treatment, and it is long past the stage where it is considered experimental.

"...In light of our current review, it is the opinion of the Medical Practice Committee that the procedure of ligament injection, known as Prolotherapy, is a clinically accepted procedure and we recommend payment of the physicians fees by the insurance company." [8]

The American Medical Association, of which the Chicago Medical Society is a local branch, is headquartered in Chicago. The Chicago Medical Society is one of the largest local branches of the AMA, and the stamp of approval was given for Prolotherapy on three separate occasions over the last 20 years.

6. IF PROLOTHERAPY IS SO EFFECTIVE, WHY IS MY DOCTOR NOT AWARE OF IT?

Prolotherapy has been presented and taught for years by the American Association of Orthopedic Medicine, the American Board of Sclerotherapy, and The George S. Hackett Foundation. (**See Appendix D, George S. Hackett AMA Presentations.**) Presentations on Prolotherapy have been given at numerous medical conferences including the First and Second Interdisciplinary World Congresses on Low Back Pain sponsored by the University of California at San Diego, "Practical Approaches to Low Back Pain" sponsored by the University of

Wisconsin Medical School, and the New Frontiers in Pain 1996 meeting. In October 1996, at the national meeting of the American Academy of Physical Medicine and Rehabilitation, K. Dean Reeves, M.D., Ed Magaziner, M.D., and Dr. Hauser presented a symposium on the treatment of chronic pain with Prolotherapy. There are many other conferences given every year on Prolotherapy for the physician desiring to learn about the treatment.

In addition to medical conferences, abundant references and research regarding Prolotherapy is available. The latest book on the different procedures used in Physical Medicine and Rehabilitation, *Physiatric Procedures,* contains a chapter devoted exclusively to Prolotherapy.[9] In addition to writing that chapter, Dr. Reeves contributed an article on Prolotherapy in a recent issue of Physical Medicine and Rehabilitation Clinics of North America.[10] William Faber, D.O., and Thomas Dorman, M.D., have written numerous articles and have published several books devoted to the treatment of chronic pain with Prolotherapy.[11, 12, 13] Physicians such as these have done their best to spread the word about Prolotherapy, but it is still relatively unknown.

Instead of asking why your doctor is not aware of Prolotherapy, give your doctor this book and ask him or her that question. Anyone involved in chronic pain management has the opportunity to learn about Prolotherapy.

7. WHY MAY PHYSICAL THERAPY, MASSAGE, AND CHIROPRACTIC MANIPULATION PROVIDE ONLY TEMPORARY RELIEF?

For the chronic pain patient, the source of the pain is most commonly due to ligament laxity. These therapies usually treat the symptoms and not the underlying cause. Physical therapy modalities such as TENS units, electrical stimulation units, massage, and ultrasound will decrease muscle spasm and permanently relieve pain if muscles are the source of the problem. The chronic pain patients' muscles are in spasm or are tense usually because the underlying joint is hypermobile, or loose, and the muscles contract in order to stabilize the joint. Chronic muscle tension and spasm is a sign that the underlying joints have ligament injury.

Manual manipulation is a very effective treatment for eliminating acute pain by realigning vertebral and bony structures. Temporary benefit after years of manipulation treatment is an indication that vertebral segments are weak because of lax ligaments. Continued manipulation will not strengthen vertebral segments. Weak vertebral ligaments are the cause of the mal-aligned vertebrae, known as subluxation.

The common source of chronic pain is loose joints, which is not resolved by manipulative treatment. However, any treatment that improves blood flow while undergoing Prolotherapy, such as massage, myofascial release, body work, ultrasound, and heat will enhance the body's response to Prolotherapy.

8. WHAT ENHANCES OR LIMITS LIGAMENT AND TENDON TISSUE HEALING?

There are many factors that are involved in a person's ability to heal after Prolotherapy. Age, obesity, hormones, nutrition, sleep, physical activity, medications, concurrent treatment regimes used, and infections are some of these factors. All of these have an effect on a person's immune function. Good immune function is needed for a person to adequately heal soft tissue injuries and respond well to Prolotherapy.

Prolotherapy initiates the growth of ligament and tendon tissue, but the body actually grows the tissue. If the body is deprived of the necessary building blocks to grow strong new tissue, the response to Prolotherapy will be reduced. Therefore all factors that decrease tendon and ligament growth should be increased before and during Prolotherapy to ensure complete healing. Prolotherapy's effectiveness and the body's ability to complete the healing process is different for each individual. [14, 15, 16, 17, 18] **(See Chapters 9 and 10 for more information.)**

9. WHAT IS THE EFFECT OF AGE ON HEALING?

We are frequently asked to speak to retirement groups and are always amazed how few people truly enjoy retirement. Marion's father retired about 15 years ago. He currently exercises three times a week, enjoys wonderful health, visits his children and grandchildren, and travels with his wife around the country. At our charity clinic in southern Illinois, he uses his work experience as a chemist to perform all of the REAMS testing. He has far more energy than most younger folks at the clinic. This is how retirement should be for everyone!

What we have seen is usually the opposite. People's faces grimacing in pain when getting up from a chair, and a body that is bent over a walker when ambulating is more typical. Unfortunately, people are forced to use canes, walkers, or wheelchairs for transportation. Some reside in nursing homes because of their ill health. We would prefer our dad's type of retirement.

It is also amazing how few people seek out Prolotherapy treatments after learning that relief from their pain is possible. It appears that the feeling among the aged is that pain is just a normal part of the aging process. There is no honor in suffering needlessly from pain.

Losing the ability to be mobile and active is possibly the worst thing that can happen to people as they age. Activity truly keeps the blood flowing. Joints like the hips and knees depend on walking and weight-bearing activities to provide nourishment to the joint cartilage. No walking, no nourishment. No nourishment, no cartilage. No cartilage, no movement. Walking keeps people alive and keeps the body functioning. If stiffness sets in, the grave may follow. **(See Figure 5-3.)**

Because most bodily functions decline with age, the ability to heal an injury and the immune system response are slower. With age, the ligament and tendon

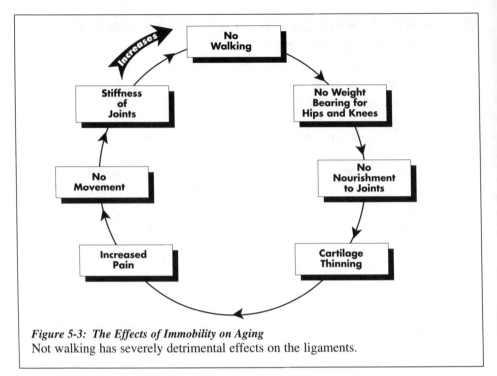

Figure 5-3: The Effects of Immobility on Aging
Not walking has severely detrimental effects on the ligaments.

tissue contain less water, noncollagenous protein, and proteoglycans. Proteoglycans are a proteinaceous material containing a large quantity of water. The proteoglycans and subcomponents, such as glucosamine and chondroitin sulfate, allow structures like ligaments, intervertebral discs, and articular cartilage to withstand intense pressure.[19, 20, 21] The collagen matrix becomes disorganized and prone to injury. Chronic ligament and tendon laxity is a reason for chronic pain in the aging population. For these reasons, older people may respond slower and because of this slower healing more Prolotherapy sessions may be needed. Teenagers, because they are in the growing phase of life, rarely need more than one Prolotherapy treatment to eliminate chronic pain. Someone in their 90's will heal slower because of their age and often require more than the typical four Prolotherapy sessions to cure their chronic pain.

Pain is not a normal part of the aging process. Chronic pain always has a cause and that cause is not old age syndrome. Chronic pain is almost always due to ligament weakness. Prolotherapy can help strengthen ligaments at any age and is the treatment of choice for chronic pain, regardless of age.

10. WHAT IS THE EFFECT OF OBESITY ON HEALING?

Ligaments, which provide stability to the joints, resist stretching (good tensile strength). Tensile strength of ligaments is much less than the tensile strength of bone. Thus, when a joint is stressed, the ligament will be injured prior to the bone because it is the weak link of the bone-ligament complex.[22] The ligament will stretch and sprain before the bone will fracture. The area where the ligament is injured is the fibro-osseous junction.

The strength of the ligament required to maintain the stability of the joint depends directly on the pressure applied. The heavier the force applied to the joint, the stronger the ligament must be to hold the joint in place. A tackle by Dick Butkus, former middle linebacker of the Chicago Bears, requires ligaments to withstand more pressure in order to maintain knee stability than being tackled by us. This explains why overweight people, exhibiting a positive "basketball-belly sign," are prone to chronic pain and impaired healing. The excess weight places increased pressure on the ligaments, especially in the lower back, hip, and knee areas. These ligaments stretch and weaken and begin the process known as osteoarthritis.

Weight loss is effective for decreasing the pain of osteoarthritis and chronic ligament and tendon weakness because it diminishes the stress on the joints. Stabilization and movement of the joint requires less work by the ligaments and tendons, resulting in reduced pain.

11. Do Hormones Play a Role In Healing?

The endocrine system produces and secretes hormones for the body, including adrenal hormones such as cortisol, thyroid hormones, growth hormone, melatonin, prostaglandins, and insulin. Hormones such as testosterone, cortisol, and thyroxine regulate the growth of tissue. An inadequate endocrine system will propagate ligament and tendon weakness. Soft tissue healing of ligaments and tendons will be compromised if any of these hormones are deficient.[23, 24, 25] Hormone levels also naturally decrease with age. Therefore, these hormones may need to be supplemented in order to ensure complete healing.

To be evaluated for hormone deficiencies and the use of natural hormones, an evaluation by a Natural Medicine physician should be considered.

12. What Is the Role of Nutrition In Healing?

Nutritional deficiencies are epidemic in modern society affecting both overall health and the healing of ligaments and tendons. Ligaments and tendons consist of water, proteoglycans, and collagen. Collagen represents 70 to 90 percent of the weight of connective tissues and is the most abundant protein in the human body, approximately 30 percent of total proteins, and six percent of human body weight.

Collagen synthesis requires specific nutrients including iron, copper, manganese, calcium, zinc, vitamin C, and various amino acids.[26] Proteoglycan synthesis requires the coordination of protein, carbohydrate polymer, and collagen synthesis, along with trace minerals such as manganese, copper, and zinc. Proper nutrition is an essential factor in soft tissue healing. A diet lacking in adequate nutrients such as vitamin A, vitamin C, zinc, and protein will hinder the healing process and the formation of collagen tissue. For these reasons, everyone should take a good multi-vitamin and mineral supplement.

It is also important that we eat an appropriate diet for our metabolism and take vitamins according to our metabolic type. **(See Appendix A, Nutrition and Chronic Pain, to learn more about Metabolic Typing.)** To assist healing after Prolotherapy, we recommend nutritional supplements which contain specific nutrients that are needed in soft tissue healing. Some of the supplements we use are from Orthomolecular Products called Ortho Prolo Max, Ortho Derma, and Cosmedix. **(See Appendix C, Natural Medicine Nutritional Products, for information.)**

Water is the most necessary nutrient in the body. The human body is composed of 25 percent solid matter and 75 percent water. Many of the supporting structures of the body, including the articular cartilage surfaces of joints and the intervertebral discs, contain a significant amount of water. Seventy-five percent of the weight of the upper part of the body is supported by the water volume stored in the disc core.[27] Inadequate intake of water may lead to inadequate fluid support to these areas, resulting in weakened structures that may produce chronic pain. In order to determine the amount of water you should drink daily, divide your body weight in pounds by two. This equals the amount of water you should drink in ounces per day. For example, a 150 pound man should drink 75 ounces of distilled, filtered water per day.

13. WHAT IS THE ROLE OF SLEEP IN HEALING?

Chronic pain patients are often prescribed anti-depressant medications like Elavil to aid sleep. These medicines provide some temporary pain relief and aid sleep. However, chronic pain is not due to an Elavil or other pharmaceutical drug deficiency. Chronic pain has a cause. Until the etiology is determined and treated, all therapeutic modalities will provide only temporary relief. Prolotherapy injections to strengthen the ligament and tendon attachments to bone cause permanent healing.

EFFECT OF CHRONIC PAIN ON CORTISOL LEVELS & SLEEP

Chronic pain leads to high cortisol levels at bedtime which results in an awake state of mind and chronic insomnia.

	PAIN-FREE	CHRONIC-PAIN
Night Cortisol Levels	Low	High
State of Mind at Bedtime	Restful	Restless
End Result	Sleep	Insomnia

Figure 5-4

Chronic pain and chronic insomnia go hand in hand. The adrenal gland secretion of the hormone cortisol normally decreases at night and the pineal gland secretion of melatonin increases, thereby enabling sleep. Unfortunately, the chronic pain patient's secretion of cortisol does not decline because chronic pain is seen by the body as stress, thereby stimulating the adrenal gland, which reacts to stress, to produce cortisol. This results in chronic insomnia. **(See Figure 5-4.)** The secretion of cortisol will stop only when the chronic pain is relieved. Chronic insomnia increases chronic pain. Prolotherapy breaks this cycle. Pain relief leads to a good night's sleep.

Sleep is vital to health maintenance. Sleep stimulates the anterior pituitary to produce growth hormone. Growth hormone is one of the main anabolic, meaning to grow or repair, hormones in the body whose job is to repair the damage done to the body during the day. Every day, soft tissues including ligaments and tendons are damaged. It is vital to obtain deep stages of sleep, as during this time growth hormone is secreted.

Without deep stages of sleep, inadequate growth hormone is secreted and soft tissue healing is inadequate. **(See Figure 5-5.)** Growth hormone levels also appear to be increased with exercise and amino acid supplementation with ornithine, arginine, or glutamine.[28, 29]

A natural way to increase sleep and improve deep sleep is aerobic exercise like cycling, walking, or running. Melatonin, L-Tryptophan (an amino acid) valerian root, and gamma hydroxybutyrate are also beneficial natural sleep aids.

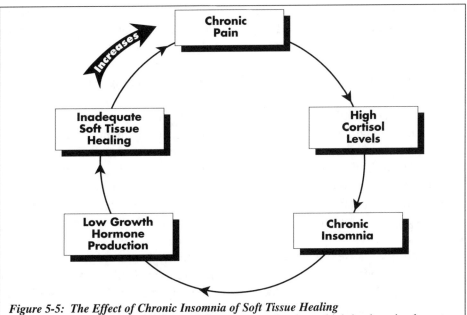

Figure 5-5: The Effect of Chronic Insomnia of Soft Tissue Healing
Chronic insomnia causes low growth hormone production which leads to inadequate soft tissue production.

14. WHAT IS THE ROLE OF PHYSICAL ACTIVITY IN HEALING?

Exercise is currently the traditional treatment of choice for chronic pain. Chronic pain patients often experience an exacerbation of their pain when exercising. This is an indication that ligament laxity is the cause of the pain. Ligament laxity generally causes pain when the joint is stressed, which occurs with activity. The proper treatment is not to "work through the pain," but to correct the source of the pain. The main function of exercise is to strengthen muscle, not to grow ligament tissue.

Aggressive exercise may worsen ligament injury and is not recommended until Prolotherapy has strengthened the joint sufficiently to provide pain relief. A good rule-of-thumb is if doing something hurts, don't do it. Doctors are smart aren't they? Once healing begins and the pain has decreased, dynamic range-of-motion exercises like walking, cycling, and swimming are more helpful than static-resistive exercises like weight-lifting.[30] A more formal exercise program is necessary after the ligaments strengthen and the joint stabilizes. This exercise program will strengthen the muscles around the joint and increase the flexibility of the muscles which protect the joint from reinjury.

15. SHOULD I IMMOBILIZE THE INJURED AREA?

Immobilization, also known as stress deprivation, is extremely detrimental to the body's joints and ligaments. Immobilization causes the following changes to occur inside joints: **1.** proliferation of fatty connective tissue within the joint, **2.** cartilage damage and necrosis, **3.** scar tissue formation and articular cartilage tears, **4.** increased randomness of the collagen fibers within the ligaments and connective tissues, and **5.** ligament weakening with a decreased resistance to stretch. [31, 32, 33]

A study performed on animals revealed that after several weeks of immobilization, the strength of the ligament tissue was reduced to about one-third of normal. [34, 35, 36, 37] Immobilization also significantly decreases the strength of the fibroosseous junction, the bone-ligament interface.[38] Eight weeks of immobilization produced a 39 percent decrease in the strength of the fibro-osseous junction of the anterior cruciate ligament of the knee.[39, 40] Other researchers have shown that even partial immobilization (restricted activity) has similar deleterious effects on ligament insertion sites.[41]

Immobility causes decreased water content, decreased proteoglycans, increased collagen turnover, and a dramatic alteration in the type of collagen cross-linking of the ligaments producing a weak ligament.[42, 43] Immobility is one of the primary reasons ligaments heal inadequately after an injury.

Unfortunately, the standard treatment for a tendon strain or ligament sprain is Rest, Ice, Compression, and Elevation, also known as RICE. Any emergency room or sports medicine book will recommend this same course of treatment. A newsletter from a local hospital recently came in the mail. It recommended the RICE treatment for an acute soft tissue injury of a ligament or tendon. This treatment is provided because the pain is relieved in the short-term. However, research reveals that the RICE treatment actually impairs healing and contributes to chronic ligament and tendon relaxation. Any treatment that impairs soft tissue healing increases the risk of incomplete ligament and tendon repair and predisposes the structure to future injury and becoming a source of chronic pain.

16. Should I Put Ice on My Injury?

As a result of immobilization (rest), ice, compression, and elevation, blood flow is decreased resulting in reduced immune cell production necessary to remove the debris from the injury site. This produces formation of weak ligament and tendon tissue. (**See Figure 5-6.**) Swelling is the physical manifestation of inflammation. Swelling is evidence that the body is working to heal itself. Use of ice will obviously prevent the body from doing its work. Ice treatment has many harmful effects. It has been shown that as little as five minutes of icing a knee can decrease both blood flow to the soft tissues and skeletal metabolism.[44] Icing an area for 25 minutes decreases blood flow and skeletal metabolism another 400 percent. Healing is hindered by a decrease in blood flow and metabolism to the area. Icing increases the chance of incomplete healing by decreasing blood flow to the injured ligaments and tendons. This increases the chance of re-injury or the development of chronic pain.

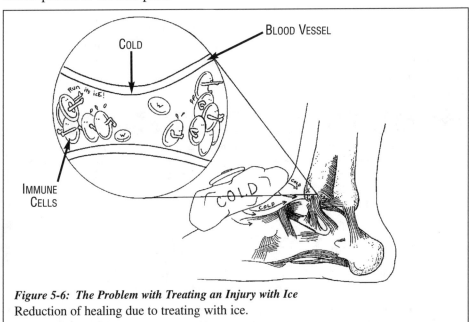

Figure 5-6: The Problem with Treating an Injury with Ice
Reduction of healing due to treating with ice.

17. Is Prolotherapy Useful for Acute Injuries?

If inflammation is so beneficial, why not use Prolotherapy for the treatment of an acute injury? Prolotherapy is beneficial and will speed the recovery process of an acute injury. However, the first treatment course should always be the most conservative one. A more conservative approach to treating acute injuries to ligaments and tendons is Movement, Exercise, Analgesics, and Treatment, also known as

MEAT. While immobility is detrimental to soft tissue healing, movement is beneficial.[45] Movement and gentle range-of-motion exercises improve blood flow to the area, removing debris. Heat also increases blood flow so this is recommended after an acute injury. If movement of the joint is painful, then isometric exercises should be performed. Isometric exercising involves contracting a muscle without movement of the affected joint. An example of this is a handshake. Both parties squeeze, creating a muscle contraction without joint movement.

Natural analgesics or pain relievers that are not synthetic anti-inflammatories may be used. Natural substances such as the enzymes Bromelain, Trypsin, and Papain aid soft tissue healing by reducing the viscosity of extracellular fluid. This increases nutrient and waste transport from the injured site, reducing swelling or edema.[46] A narcotic such as codeine may be prescribed short term for an extremely painful acute injury. Narcotics are wonderful pain relievers and do not interfere with the natural healing mechanisms of the body, if used in the short-term. Your body produces its own narcotics, called endorphins, which work to reduce pain from an acute injury. Other options for pain control include Tylenol or Ultram. As previously mentioned, these can be used as they relieve pain but do not decrease inflammation.

The "T" in MEAT stands for specific Treatments that increase blood flow and immune cell migration to the damaged area which will aid in ligament and tendon healing. Treatments such as physical therapy, massage, chiropractic care, ultrasound, myofascial release, and electrical stimulation all improve blood flow and assist soft tissue healing. **(See Figure 5-7.)**

RICE VS MEAT

The RICE protocol hampers soft tissue healing whereas MEAT encourages healing.

	RICE	MEAT
Immune System Response	Decreased	Increased
Blood Flow to Injured Area	Decreased	Increased
Collagen Formation	Hindered	Encouraged
Speed of Recovery	Delayed (lengthened)	Hastened (shortened)
Range of Motion of Joint	Decreased	Increased
Complete Healing	Decreased	Increased

Figure 5-7

If circumstances are such that time is a factor, some Prolotherapy physicians will use Prolotherapy as an initial treatment for acute pain. Rodney Van Pelt, M.D., is one Prolotherapist who utilizes Prolotherapy in the management of acute sports injury. An athlete who would normally wait two to three months for an acute injury to heal may heal in only two to three weeks if given Prolotherapy. Dr. Van Pelt has seen this increased speed of recovery in a multitude of sports injuries including ACL (anterior cruciate ligament) sprains of the knee. We have seen the same results in our office. The late David Brewer, M.D., who was an obstetrician and gynecologist, used Prolotherapy in the treatment of low back pain of pregnancy. This safe and effective treatment is extremely helpful in relieving the low back pain experienced during and after pregnancy.

18. CAN I TAKE ANTI-INFLAMMATORY AGENTS?

Anti-inflammatory medicines, like Motrin, Advil, aspirin, Clinoril, Volteran, Prednisone, and Cortisone, all inhibit the healing process of soft tissues. The long-term detrimental effects far outweigh the temporary positive effect of decreased pain. Aspirin does have a beneficial effect on the heart, but a detrimental effect on soft tissue healing. When a ligament or tendon is injured, prostaglandins are released which initiate vasodilation in noninjured blood vessels. This enables healthy blood vessels to increase blood flow and immune cell flow to the injured area to begin the repair process. The use of anti-inflammatories inhibits the release of prostaglandins thus ultimately decreasing the blood flow to the injured area.[47]

As previously stated, nonsteroidal anti-inflammatory drugs (NSAIDs) have been shown to produce short-term pain benefit but leave long-term loss of function.[48] NSAIDs also inhibit proteoglycan synthesis, a component of ligament and cartilage tissue. Proteoglycans are essential for the elasticity and compressive stiffness of articular cartilage and suppression of their synthesis has significant adverse effects on the joint.[49, 50, 51]

NSAID prescription for acute soft tissue injury is considered standard practice. The administration of NSAIDs, in combination with the RICE treatment, nearly eliminates the body's ability to heal. Is it any wonder so many people live with chronic pain? In our opinion, the current medical treatment for acute soft tissue injuries is contributing to this epidemic.

NSAIDs are the mainstay treatment for acute ligament and tendon injuries, yet efficacy in their usefulness is lacking.[52] Worse yet is the long-term use by people with chronic pain. Studies in the use of NSAIDs for chronic hip pain revealed an acceleration of arthritis in the people taking NSAIDs.[53, 54, 55]

In one study, NSAID use was associated with progressive formation of multiple small acetabular and femoral subcortical cysts and subchondral bone thinning. In this study, 84 percent of the people who had progressive arthritis were long-term NSAID users. The conclusion of the study was "this highly significant association between NSAID use and acetabular destruction gives cause for concern."[56] As it should, acetabular destruction, femoral subcortical cysts, and subchondral bone thinning are all signs that the NSAIDs were causing arthritis to form more quickly. This is one explanation why people taking Motrin, Advil, Voltaren, or any other NSAID will likely require more medicine to decrease their pain. Eventually the medicine does not stop the pain because the arthritis process

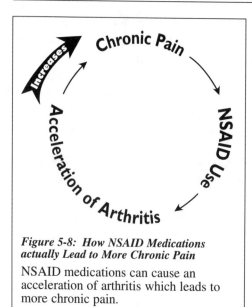

Figure 5-8: How NSAID Medications actually Lead to More Chronic Pain

NSAID medications can cause an acceleration of arthritis which leads to more chronic pain.

is actually accelerating while taking the medicine. **(See Figure 5-8.)**

The end result of taking NSAIDs for pain relief is an arthritic joint. How many times has Motrin or any other NSAID cured a person of his or her pain? Prolotherapy eliminates the cause of chronic pain and often cures the person's pain. Even long-term aspirin use has been associated with accelerating hip damage from arthritis.[57] When comparing the long-term use of Indomethacin in the treatment of osteoarthritis of the hip it was clearly shown that the disease progressed more frequently and the destruction within the hip joint was more severe with drug use than without.[58]

For women of child-bearing age who want to have children but have pain, Prolotherapy is a better choice for another reason.[59] NSAIDs have caused concern that they may be associated with an increased rate of infertility in females because they delay the egg from being released. NSAIDs are truly anti-inflammatory in their mechanism of action. Since all tissues heal by inflammation, one can see why long-term use of these medications will have harmful effects. Osteoarthritis and other chronic pain disorders are not an Indomethacin or other NSAID deficiency. This is why the use of these drugs will never cure any disease. Their chronic long-term use will not cure, and will hamper soft tissue healing and accelerate the arthritic process.

Prolotherapy, because it stimulates inflammation, helps the body heal itself. Prolotherapy stops the arthritic process and helps eliminate the person's chronic pain, often permanently. NSAIDs should not be taken while undergoing Prolotherapy because they inhibit the inflammation caused by the treatment. For that matter, anyone with chronic pain should seriously consider stopping NSAIDs and starting Prolotherapy.

19. WHAT ABOUT STEROID INJECTIONS?

The next assault to the already weakened ligament and tendon tissue after RICE and NSAID treatments is the steroid injection. The unfortunate person who has been subjected to RICE and NSAID treatments will likely be offered a steroid injection for the pain which has now become chronic. The RICE-and NSAID-weakened ligament and tendon will be further attacked by each subsequent steroid injection. A cyclical pattern of injury, improper treatment, further

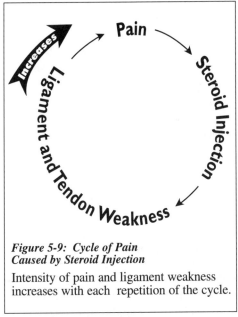

Figure 5-9: Cycle of Pain Caused by Steroid Injection

Intensity of pain and ligament weakness increases with each repetition of the cycle.

injury, and ultimately, chronic pain, emerges. This leads to further weakness in the tissue and the cycle repeats itself. **(See Figure 5-9.)**

Corticosteroids, such as Cortisone and Prednisone, have an adverse effect on bone and soft tissue healing. Corticosteroids inactivate vitamin D, limiting calcium absorption by the gastrointestinal tract and increasing urinary excretion of calcium. Bone also shows a decrease in calcium uptake, ultimately leading to weakness at the fibro-osseous junction. Corticosteroids also inhibit the release of growth hormone which further decreases soft tissue and bone repair. Ultimately, corticosteroids lead to a decrease in bone, ligament, and tendon strength.[60, 61, 62, 63, 64, 65]

Corticosteroids inhibit the synthesis of proteins, collagen, and proteoglycans in articular cartilage, by inhibiting chondrocyte production, the cells that comprise the articular cartilage. The net catabolic effect (weakening) of corticosteroids is inhibition of fibroblast production of collagen, ground substance, and angiogenesis (new blood vessel formation). The result is weakened synovial joints, supporting structures, and ligaments and tendons. This weakness increases pain and the increased pain leads to more steroid injections. Corticosteroids should not be used as a treatment for chronic pain due to ligament and tendon weakness. The treatment of choice for such conditions is Prolotherapy.

20. WHAT IS pH AND HOW DOES IT AFFECT HEALING?

We utilize a simple diagnostic testing procedure known as Metabolic Typing to determine a person's underlying physiology.[66, 67] **(See Appendix A, Nutrition and Chronic Pain, for more information on Metabolic Typing.)** The test consists of, among other things, determining blood, urine, and saliva pH. The tests consistently reveal that chronic pain patients suffer from chronic dehydration. Chronic dehydration produces a reduction in shock absorbing capabilities of the intervertebral discs and articular cartilage, placing additional stress on the ligaments to stabilize the joints. The end result is ligament laxity, injury, and resultant chronic pain. **(See Figure 5-10.)** It is very important for the person in chronic pain to drink six to eight glasses of purified water per day.

A significant number of chronic pain patients also have a lower than normal venous blood plasma pH.[68] A person with low venous plasma pH has what is

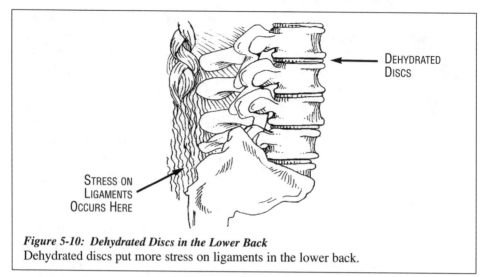

Figure 5-10: Dehydrated Discs in the Lower Back
Dehydrated discs put more stress on ligaments in the lower back.

termed acid blood. Acid blood is typically dark in color due to low oxygen content. Oxygen is the food that allows the body to extract and store energy from the blood. A low oxygen content in the blood compromises healing capabilities.

The treatment for acid blood is to consume foods and supplements which neutralize the blood pH. This is accomplished by consuming items which are alkaline and by reducing the intake of acidic items. Caffeine, sugar, wheat, citrus fruits, soda pop, and potatoes should be avoided, whereas protein and vegetables should be the majority of the meal. Supplements such as green algae or alfalfa also help neutralize acidic blood. A diet similar to that discussed by Barry Sears, Ph.D. in the book *The Zone* works very well.[69] Nuts, seeds, brown rice, or soy products are good sources of protein if a vegetarian diet is preferred. People with acid blood are typically carbohydrate addicts and consume very little protein. Protein is needed in the diet because collagen, which makes up ligaments and tendons, is the most abundant protein in the body. Collagen is the building block for ligament and tendon tissue. A healthy diet with adequate amounts of protein for soft tissue growth is essential for healing ligament and tendon injuries. (**See Appendix A, Nutrition and Chronic Pain.**)

21. Does Chronic Infection Affect Healing?

Chronic pain patients commonly possess a myriad of other conditions including diabetes, allergies, and fungal and sinus infections. The immune system's primary function is to sustain life. If chronic sinus or fungal infection exists, the immune system will preferentially fight these conditions versus healing a ligament or tendon injury. Controlling all infections, allergies, or other chronic health problems is essential to healing chronic ligament or tendon injury. We prefer to use natural treatments like garlic, echinacea, tea tree oil, and goldenseal to fight infections. Facial dipping which cleanses the nose is helpful for allergies. The nose is a

62

filter and should be cleansed periodically. Facial dipping involves dipping the face in an iodine-salt-water mixture and breathing it up into the nostrils. It works great! Natural botanicals such as stinging nettles, curcumin, and quercetin also decrease allergic symptoms. **(See Appendix C, Natural Medicine Nutritional Products.)** This is one of the reasons that anyone with chronic pain should see a Prolotherapist, as most Prolotherapists also practice Natural Medicine.

22. WHAT IS THE ROLE OF IMMUNE FUNCTION IN HEALING?

All of the above reasons for inadequate soft tissue healing have one thing in common, they all lead to suboptimal immune function. Immune function declines with age, and endocrine or nutritional inadequacies. Immobility, RICE, NSAIDs, infections, allergies, acid blood, and poor tissue oxygenation all cause a decline in the immune response. This poor immune response causes poor ligament and tissue healing, resulting in chronic pain. Chronic pain may lead to immobility and subsequent use of NSAIDs, which leads to insomnia and depression, which causes some people to eat "lousy" (or at least gives them an excuse), which can lead to acid blood and poor tissue oxygenation, producing further tissue and tendon weakness. There is only one thing that can break this cycle: Prolotherapy.

If these above issues are addressed, a person who has chronic pain as a result of ligament or tendon injury has an excellent prognosis for complete healing with Prolotherapy. ■

CHAPTER 6

Prolotherapy, Inflammation and Healing: What's the Connection?

D uring Ross's fourth year of medical school, on a dermatology rotation with four other medical students, he had the opportunity to train under Gary Solomon, M.D., one of the most respected dermatologists in the country. Dr. Solomon told the class he was going to provide the secret to understanding human disease. If we knew the secret we would be leaps and bounds ahead of our colleagues and be masterful clinicians. Ross couldn't wait to hear it!

When that day finally arrived, Dr. Solomon explained that *inflammation* was the most important concept to understanding health and healing, especially in regard to the etiology and treatment of human ailments. Most clinicians do not understand inflammation, he said.

Inflammation?! E-Gads! Everyone knows about inflammation. At that time, Ross dismissed his comments and left disappointed. Years later when he learned about Prolotherapy, he realized Dr. Solomon had been right. Inflammation is the mechanism by which the body heals, regardless of the illness.

AN OLYMPIC-SIZE EXAMPLE

Kerri Strug became the heroine of the 1996 Summer Olympics by "sticking" her final vault to secure a gold medal for the American team in women's gymnastics. The most dramatic aspect of this vault was that she flew through the air and landed on a badly sprained ankle. As she lay wincing in pain after her heroic vault, she was mauled by medical personnel.

Unfortunately, she was observed throughout the rest of the Olympics with her ankle wrapped and her foot elevated. "What will happen to Kerri Strug? Will she finish the competition?" viewers wondered. "Will she be left with a weak ankle? Will she have chronic pain?" If the medical treatment she received at the Olympics is any indication, she will be anti-inflaming her pain to stay.

Kerri Strug suffered a ligament sprain. Ligaments are the supporting structures of the musculoskeletal system that connect the bones to each other. A stretched and weakened ligament is defined as a sprain.

Immediately after her ligament injury, Kerri Strug was given the currently accepted mode of treatment known as RICE. This treatment is prescribed by most physicians, athletic trainers, physical therapists, and chiropractors for an acute injury of a ligament or tendon. The treatment consists of Rest, Ice, Compression, and Elevation in order to immobilize the joint and decrease the swelling. The short-term result of this treatment is a reduction in pain. For the treatment of soft tissue injury, however, the RICE treatment decreases blood flow preventing immune cells from getting to the injured area. This impairs the healing process, causes greater pain long-term, and increases the chance of incomplete healing of the injured ligament. **(See Figure 6-1.)**

RICE VS MEAT

The RICE treatment leads to incomplete healing of soft tissue whereas MEAT encourages complete healing.

MODALITY	RESULT	MODALITY	RESULT
REST	Decreased joint nutrition	**M**OVEMENT	Increased joint nutrition
ICE	Decreased blood flow	**E**XERCISE	Increased blood flow
COMPRESSION	Decreased pain control	**A**NALGESIC	Increased pain control
ELEVATION	Incomplete healing	**T**REATMENT	Complete healing

Figure 6-1: RICE Versus MEAT

WHERE COMPLETE HEALING BEGINS

All human ailments, including ligament and tendon injury, involve inflammation. Inflammation is defined as the reaction of vascularized living tissue to local injury.[1] The first stage of inflammation is the actual injury. Inflammation is the body's reaction to a local injury. Healing an injured area is dependent on the blood supplying inflammatory cells to repair the damaged tissue, which explains why vascularized living tissue is crucial to the repair of any injured area. Vascularization refers to the blood supply to an area. Poor blood flow proportionately reduces healing.

Chronically weak ligaments and tendons are a result of inadequate repair following an injury and occur because of poor blood supply to the area where ligaments and tendons attach to the bone, the fibro-osseous junction.[2, 3, 4] **(See Figure 6-2.)** Due to the poor blood supply, the immune cells necessary to repair the affected area cannot reach the injury. Inadequate healing is the result. Nonsteroidal anti-inflammatory drugs (NSAIDs) and ice treatments decrease the blood flow even further thus hampering the body's capability to heal the injured tissue.

Healing of an injured tissue, such as a ligament, progresses through a series of stages: inflammatory, fibroblastic, and maturation.[5, 6, 7] The inflammatory stage is characterized by an increase in blood flow transporting healing immune cells to the area, often resulting in painful swelling. Swelling tells the body, especially the brain, that an area of the body has been injured. The immune system is activated to send immune cells, called polymorphonuclear cells, also known as polys, to the

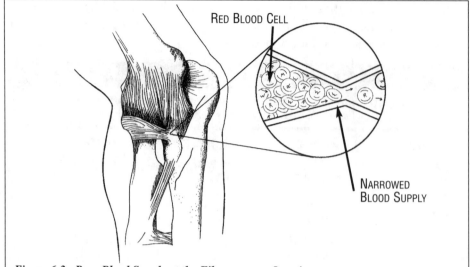

Figure 6-2: Poor Blood Supply at the Fibro-osseous Junction
The fibro-osseous junction normally has poor blood supply compared to other structures such as muscles.

injured area and remove the debris. **(See Figure 6-3.)** Other immune cells including the monocytes, histocytes, and macrophage cells assist in the cleanup. The macrophages and polys begin the process of phagocytosis, also called dinner, whereby they engulf and subsequently destroy debris and any other foreign matter in the body.

A day or two after the initial injury, the fibroblastic stage of healing begins. The body forms new blood vessels, a process called angiogenesis, because of fac-

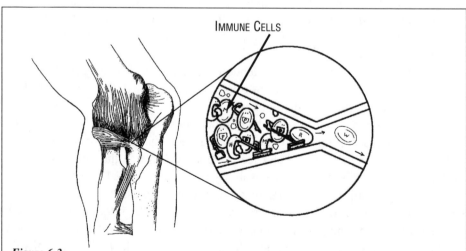

Figure 6-3:
Immune System Activity at the Fibro-osseous Junction Immediately after an Injury
Responding to an injury, the immune system activates to remove debris.

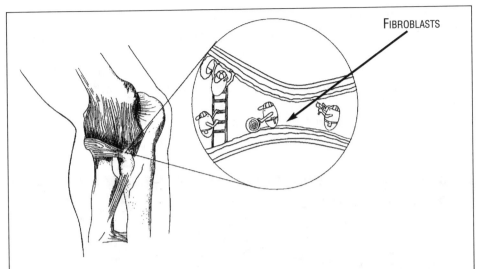

FIBROBLASTS

Figure 6-4: Immune System growing Tissue at the Fibro-osseous Junction
Fibroblasts forming new collagen tissue which makes the ligament and tendon strong.

tors released by the macrophage cells. Fibroblasts are formed from local cells or other immune cells in the blood. They are the carpenters of the body which form new collagen tissue, the building blocks of ligaments and tendons. **(See Figure 6-4.)** Collagen is responsible for the strength of the ligament and tendon. The fibroblastic stage continues for approximately six weeks after the injury. Consequently, Prolotherapy treatments are administered every six weeks, allowing maximal time for ligament and tendon growth.[8]

The maturation phase of healing begins after the fibroblastic stage and may continue for 18 months after an injury. During this time the collagen fibers increase in density and diameter, resulting in increased strength. **(See Figure 6-5.)**

THREE STAGES OF HEALING			
	INFLAMMATION	**FIBROBLASTIC**	**MATURATION**
Effect on blood	Increased blood flow	Formation of new blood vessels	New blood vessels mature
Symptoms	Swelling and pain increase	Swelling and pain subside	If tissue is strong, pain subsides
Physiology	Immune cells called macrophages remove damaged tissue	Immune cells called fibroblasts form new collagen	Increased density and diameter of collagen fibers occur if healing is not hindered
Length of time	Immediate response occurs for a week	Begins at day 2 or 3 after injury and continues for 6 weeks	Continues from day 42 until 18 months after injury

Figure 6-5: Three Stages of Healing After Soft Tissue Injury

Anything that decreases inflammation is detrimental to the healing process of soft tissue injury. NSAIDs, for example, should only be prescribed when inflammation is the cause of the problem. In the case of soft tissue injury, inflammation is the cure for the problem. Prolotherapy injections stimulate ligament and tendon tissue growth, which only occurs through the process of inflammation. Dr. Solomon was indeed right. Inflammation is the key to the treatment of human ailments. Those who suffer from chronic pain have a choice: Anti-inflame the pain to stay or inflame your pain away with Prolotherapy. ■

PROLOTHERAPY STIMULATES INFLAMMATION

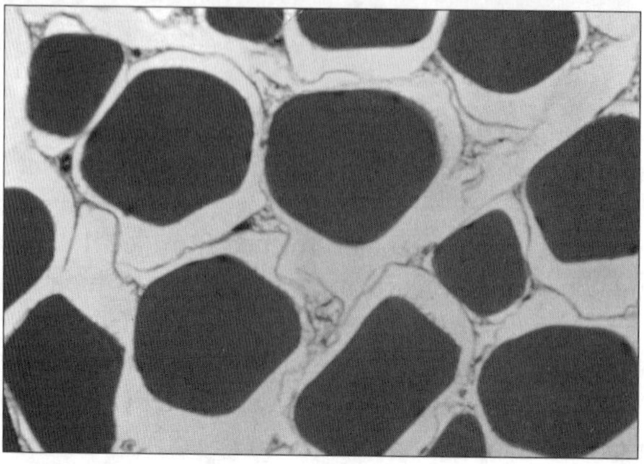

NORMAL MUSCLE TISSUE

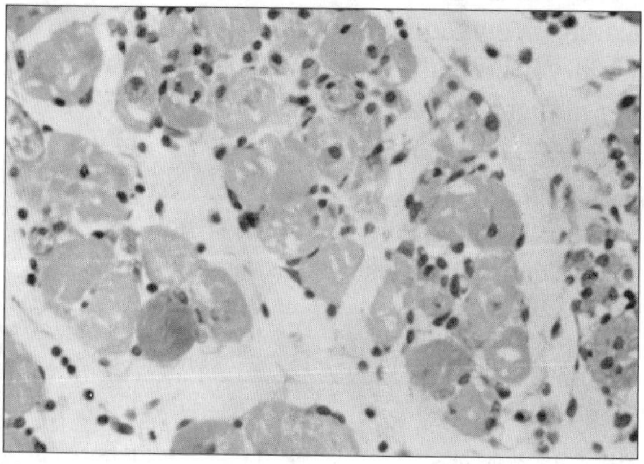

MUSCLE TISSUE 48 HOURS AFTER PROLOTHERAPY:
Injections with 12.5% Dextrose in 0.5% Xylocaine. Notice the massive inflammatory reaction—the basis of Prolotherapy

Slides prepared by Gale Bordon, M.D., from K. Dean Reeves, M.D. Used with permission.

Figure 6-6: Prolotherapy Stimulates Inflammation
Prolotherapy stimulates the natural healing mechanisms of the body via inflammation.

CHAPTER 7

Prolo Your Back Pain Away!

Baseball has its original iron man, Lou Gehrig and more recently Cal Ripken, but hockey's iron man will always be Stan Mikita of the Chicago Blackhawks. For 22 seasons, Stan dazzled hockey fans. His hockey career extended over four decades, from 1958 to 1980, during which time he amassed 1,467 total points, played in 18 playoff series, and was a member of the 1961 Stanley Cup championship team. Stan Mikita is truly an iron man.

But Stan did not feel like an iron man six weeks before the 1971-72 training camp. He had such excruciating back pain that he could not even get out of bed. Stan had learned to deal with constant back pain since injuring his back during a game in the 1960s. He had sought treatment from the Mayo Clinic and some of the best sports clinics and rehabilitation specialists without success.

"I knew something had to be done. I couldn't get out of bed," Stan said. "I had heard about Dr. Hemwall's Prolotherapy treatments and decided to give it a try." Gustav A. Hemwall, M.D., the world's most experienced Prolotherapist, treated Stan's lower back twice in three weeks. Aggressive treatment was given because Stan had to report to training camp.

"The results were unbelievable!" Stan exclaimed. "For the last eight years of my career I was completely pain free. I'd say Prolotherapy definitely helped prolong my career." In 1983, Stan was elected to the National Hockey League Hall of Fame.

LIMITATIONS OF MRI AND CAT SCANS

Most medical physicians rely too heavily on diagnostic tests, especially for low back problems. Consequently, many who suffer from low back pain do not find relief. The typical scenario is as follows: A person complains to a physician about low back pain that radiates down the leg. The physician orders x-rays and a CAT or MRI scan. The MRI scan reveals an abnormality in the disc such as a herniated, bulging, or degenerated disc. Unfortunately for the patient, this finding usually has nothing to do with the pain. As discussed in Chapter Two, 50 percent of people over age 40 who are asymptomatic have such findings on a CAT scan.

In the 1980s, modern medicine developed another high-tech diagnostic tool to look at vertebrae, nerves, and discs on film—the MRI scan. Again, the same types of abnormalities were found in the vertebral discs and bones. People were subjected to various treatments and surgeries for these "abnormalities" in the hopes of curing their pain. Very few people were cured. But all received hefty bills for the tests and surgeries.

Ten years of using MRI technology passed before research was conducted on the MRI findings of the lower back of people who had no pain symptoms.[1,2] Scott Boden, M.D., found that nearly 100 percent of the people he tested who were over

60 years of age with no symptoms had abnormal findings in their lumbar spines (lower back) on MRI scans. Thirty-six percent had herniated discs and all but one had degeneration or bulging of a disc in at least one lumbar level. In the age group of 20 to 39, 35 percent had degeneration or bulging of a disc in at least one lumbar level.[3]

In a study published in *The New England Journal of Medicine* in 1994, Maureen Jensen, M.D., and associates, studied MRI scans of the lumbar spine in 98 asymptomatic people. Only 36 percent had a normal scan, 64 percent had abnormal findings overall, and 38 percent had abnormal findings in more than one lumbar vertebral level. The conclusion was "because bulges and protrusions on MRI scans in people with low back pain or even radiculopathy may be coincidental, a patient's clinical situation must be carefully evaluated in conjunction with the results of MRI studies."[4] In other words, physicians should begin listening with their ears and poking with their thumbs! X-ray studies should never take the place of a good history and physical examination. Unfortunately for many, x-ray findings have nothing to do with their pain.

DIAGNOSIS OF LOW BACK PAIN

Low back pain is one of the easiest conditions to treat with Prolotherapy. Ninety-five percent of low back pain is located in a 6-by-4 inch area, the weakest link in the vertebral-pelvis complex. At the end of the spine, four structures connect in a very small space which happens to be the 6-by-4 inch area. The fifth lumbar vertebrae connects with the base of the sacrum. This is held together by the lumbosacral ligaments. The sacrum is connected on its sides to the ilium and iliac crest. This is held together by the sacroiliac ligaments. The lumbar vertebrae is held to the iliac crest and ilium by the iliolumbar ligaments. This is typically the area treated with Prolotherapy for chronic low back pain. **(See Figure 7-1.)**

The diagnosis of ligament laxity in the lower back can be made relatively easily. Typical referral pain patterns are elicited as previously described in **Figures 2-2 to 2-5.** The sacroiliac ligaments refer pain down the posterior thigh and the lateral foot.[5, 6] The sacrotuberous and sacrospinous ligaments refer pain to the heel. The iliolumbar ligament refers pain into the groin or vagina. Iliolumbar ligament sprain should be considered for any unexplained vaginal, testicular, or groin pain.

The first step in determining ligament laxity or instability is by physical examination.[7] The examination involves maneuvering the patient into various stretched positions. If weak ligaments exist, the stressor maneuver will cause pain. Do this simple test at home: Lie flat on your back and lift your legs together as straight and as high as you can, then lower your legs. If it is more painful to lower your legs than to raise them, laxity in the lumbosacral ligaments is likely. The next step is palpating various ligaments with the thumb to elicit tenderness. A positive "jump sign" indicates ligament laxity. **(Refer to Figure 3-5.)**

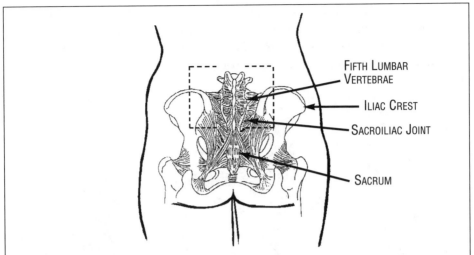

Figure 7-1: Almost All Chronic Pain in the Lower Back Occurs in a 6-by-4 Inch Area
Pain in the lower back occurs in the area where the lumbar vertebrae joins the
sacrum and iliac crest.

TREATMENT OF LOW BACK PAIN

The most common cause of unresolved chronic low back pain is injury to the
sacroiliac ligaments which typically occurs from bending over and twisting with
the knees in a locked, extended position. This maneuver stretches the sacroiliac
ligaments, placing them in a vulnerable position.

How effective is Prolotherapy in relieving chronic low back pain? In one of his
original papers, George S. Hackett, M.D., noted 82 percent of people treated for
posterior sacroiliac ligament relaxation considered themselves cured and
remained so 12 years later.[8]

HERNIATED AND DEGENERATED DISC

A herniated disc is a common diagnosis given to patients by their doctors. A
person with a degenerated, bulging, or herniated disc must realize that this may be
a coincidental finding and unrelated to the actual pain a person is experiencing. A
degenerated disc is one that is losing water and flattening. This is a usual phe-
nomenon that occurs with age. It is also normal for a disc to bulge with bending.
A herniated disc occurs when the annulus fibrosus no longer holds the gelatinous
solution in the disc. The result is a weakened disc. The annulus fibrosus is basi-
cally a ring of ligament tissue. What is the best treatment to strengthen ligament
tissue? That's right... Prolotherapy.

Why did the disc degenerate in the first place? Degeneration of a disc begins
as soon as the lumbar ligaments become loose. Once they loosen and weaken, the
vertebral segments move excessively and cause pain. The body attempts to correct
this by tensing the back muscles. Visits to a chiropractor or medical physician typ-

71

ically begin at this time. The hypermobile vertebral segments add strain to the vertebral discs. Eventually these discs cannot sustain the added pressure and begin to flatten and/or herniate. **(See Figure 7-2)** The lumbar ligaments then work harder because the discs no longer cushion the back. A dismal, downward path of pain is the end result.

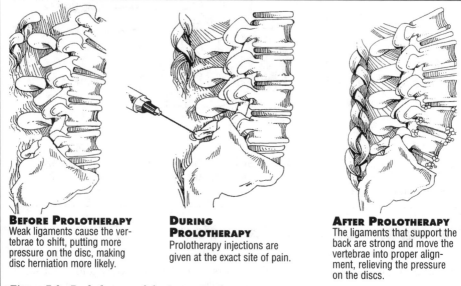

BEFORE PROLOTHERAPY
Weak ligaments cause the vertebrae to shift, putting more pressure on the disc, making disc herniation more likely.

DURING PROLOTHERAPY
Prolotherapy injections are given at the exact site of pain.

AFTER PROLOTHERAPY
The ligaments that support the back are strong and move the vertebrae into proper alignment, relieving the pressure on the discs.

Figure 7-2: Prolotherapy of the Lower Back
Prolotherapy stimulates the growth of soft tissues, such as ligaments and tendons, relieving chronic back pain.

Prolotherapy is the treatment of choice to strengthen the lumbar vertebral ligaments and prevent the progressive degeneration that occurs with age to the intervertebral discs. Prolotherapy will cause ligament and tendon growth regardless of age. Prolotherapy patients in our office range from four years of age to 94 years of age. Children and adolescents usually require only one Prolotherapy treatment to resolve a ligament or tendon injury. The young body is already primed to grow new tissue, making Prolotherapy treatments extremely effective.

Adults and the elderly may require more treatments because they are not in the growth mode of life. An adult being treated for chronic pain will receive an average of four to six sessions of Prolotherapy per area. Those with excellent immune systems will grow more ligament and tendon tissue per session and will therefore require fewer sessions. Those with poor immune systems, especially smokers, require more than the average four sessions. The Prolotherapy treatments are generally given every six weeks to allow the treated area ample time to grow strong ligaments and tendons.

A patient with chronic low back pain is typically treated with Prolotherapy injections into the insertions of the lumbosacral, iliolumbar, and sacroiliac ligaments. The initial assessment may reveal that the chronic low back pain and referred leg pain may be caused by a referred pain from other areas such as the pubic symphysis, hip joint, ischial tuberosity, sacrospinous, and sacrotuberous ligaments. Therefore these areas are also examined.

Off-centered low back pain is often caused by a posterior hip sprain or osteoarthritis of the hip. The hip joint often refers pain to the groin and down the leg to the big toe. Prolotherapy is very effective in this area, often alleviating the necessity for hip replacement surgery.

THE ROLE OF SURGERY

Except in a life-threatening situation or impending neurologic injury, surgery should always be a last resort and done only after all conservative treatments have been exhausted. Pain is not a life-threatening situation. It can be very anxiety-provoking, life-demeaning, and aggravating. Pain should not be an automatic indication that surgery is necessary. Conservative treatments such as vitamins, herbs, massage, physical therapy, chiropractic/osteopathic care, medications, and, of course, Prolotherapy should precede any surgical intervention. Conservative care for back pain is complete only after treatment with Prolotherapy.

It is not uncommon for patients to say that surgery has been recommended to resolve their painful back condition. Reasons for surgery may be herniated discs, compressed nerves, spinal stenosis, severe arthritis, and intractable pain. Such conditions may have nothing to do with the problem causing the pain. As previously discussed, abnormalities noted on an MRI scan such as a pinched nerve or herniated disc rarely are the reasons we find for someone's chronic back pain. We find at Caring Medical that ligament weakness is the number one reason for chronic low back pain, and this diagnosis is not made by an x-ray. It must be made by taking a thorough history and poking the loose ligaments and looking for a positive "jump sign."

Trying conservative treatments before undergoing surgery is only common sense. Surgery is fraught with many potential risks, one being the required anesthesia. General anesthesia greatly stresses the body and complications may occur while under, including kidney and liver failure or a heart attack. A significant percentage of anesthesia-related deaths result from the aspiration (swallowing) of food particles, foreign bodies like dentures, blood, gastric acid, oropharyngeal secretions, or bile during induction of general anesthesia.[9] Other possible complications include damage to the mouth, throat, vocal cords, or lungs from the insertion of the anesthesia tube. If you have ever seen anyone after anesthesia, you know it's no Sunday picnic!

In more than 95 percent of our patients, the true diagnosis causing the pain is different than the diagnosis the patients had been previously given. Rarely will a physician describe a ligament or tendon injury as a cause of chronic pain. Remember, ligaments and tendons often do not appear on x-rays. The diagnosis of ligament or tendon weakness cannot be made by a blood test, electrical test, or x-ray. It must be made using a listening ear and a strong thumb.

Even back in early 1981 as new and more effective methods of conservative treatments were being used (including Prolotherapy), the need for surgery was decreasing. Bernard E. Finneson, M.D., pointed out in a survey of surgical cases that "80 percent that should not... have been brought to surgery." It is quite possible that with the widespread use of Prolotherapy this percentage would be even higher.[10]

In more than 95 percent of pain cases, surgery can be avoided by utilizing Prolotherapy. Dr. Hemwall, having treated more than 10,000 pain patients, resorted to surgery for resolving a chronic pain complaint in only one percent of the patients. Our experience has been similar. In the event that surgery is necessary, the previous Prolotherapy treatment will not hinder the subsequent surgical procedure. Prolotherapy causes normal ligament and tendon tissue to form. The surgeon will observe an area treated with Prolotherapy containing strengthened ligament and tendon tissue.

PINCHED OR COMPRESSED NERVES

Another cause of back pain, although rare, may be a pinched or compressed nerve. A wonderful conservative treatment for this condition is chiropractic/osteopathic manipulation. These therapies have a high success rate for acutely compressed nerve cases because bony malalignment (subluxation) of the vertebrae is often the reason the nerve is pinched.

Why did the vertebral bones slip out of alignment? The answer is ligament laxity which causes the vertebrae to slip out of place and pinch the nerve. Nerve blocks utilizing a 70.0 percent Sarapin and 0.6 percent Lidocaine solution are often given, in addition to Prolotherapy, for this condition. This solution will relax the nerve, providing pain relief, while Prolotherapy grows ligament tissue. Upon nerve relaxation, the vertebrae will realign and the nerve compression will cease. A series of Prolotherapy treatments along with nerve blocks will usually resolve the pain. (See Figure 7-3.)

People considering surgery should exhaust all conservative treatments, including Prolotherapy, before succumbing to surgical intervention. Surgery removes tissue. Prolotherapy repairs tissue. The discs, the bones, and the joints are there for a reason. Surgical procedures removing tissue in an attempt to alleviate lower back pain will almost always leave a long-term detrimental effect on the body. Surgery ultimately makes the body weaker by removing tissue, whereas Prolotherapy makes the body stronger by growing tissue.

PROLOTHERAPY VERSUS SURGERY: A STUDY

In 1964, John R. Merriman, M.D., compared Prolotherapy versus operative fusion in the treatment of instability of the spine and pelvis and wrote, "The pur-

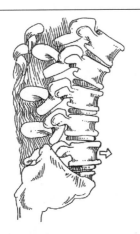 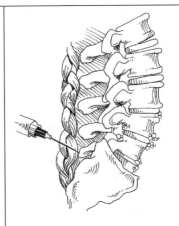

FIG. 7-3A: SPONDYLOLISTHESIS OR SUBLUXATION OF THE LOWER BACK
Weakened ligaments cause vertebrae to slip, which could lead to pinching of a nerve.

FIG. 7-3B: AFTER PROLOTHERAPY ALL THE VERTEBRAE HAVE PROPER ALIGNMENT
The proper alignment of vertebrae relieves nerve pinching.

Figure 7-3

pose of this article is to evaluate the merit of two methods of treating instability of the spine and pelvis, with which I have been concerned during 40 years as a general and industrial surgeon... The success of either method depends on regeneration of bone cells to provide joint stabilization, elimination of pain and resumption of activity... Ligament and tendon relaxation occurs when the fibro-osseous attachments to bone do not regain their normal tensile strength after sprain and lacerations, and when the attachments are weakened by decalcification from disease, menopause and aging." [11]

The figure below describes Dr. Merriman's results:[12]

AREAS EFFECTED	RESPONSE TO PROLOTHERAPY (PHYSIOLOGIC TREATMENT)	RESPONSE TO FUSION OPERATION (MECHANICAL TREATMENT)
NEW BONE	PROMPT	RETARDED
LIGAMENTS	STRENGTHENED	EXCISED (REMOVED)
TENDONS	STRENGTHENED	INCISED (CUT)
SPINOUS PROCESS	STRENGTHENED	SACRIFICED
JOINT MOTION	PRESERVED	ABOLISHED
PAIN	ELIMINATED	MAY CONTINUE
LOSS OF TIME	NEGLIGIBLE	CONSIDERABLE
RESULTS	80-90 PERCENT CURES	VARIABLE

Dr. Merriman summarized that conservative physiologic treatment by Prolotherapy after a confirmed diagnosis of ligamental and tendinous relaxation was successful in 80 to 90 percent of more than 15,000 patients treated.

TYPES OF BACK SURGERY

1. LAMINECTOMY

The most common back surgery is a laminectomy. This surgical procedure involves removing some of the bone, called lamina, from the supporting structure of the back. Its removal creates stress on other areas of the lumbar spine.

Because some of the lamina are removed, the discs, ligaments, and muscles have to do more work. As a result, the vertebral discs degenerate. The vertebral segments then move closer together and eventually become hypermobile. Back muscles tense to stabilize the segment. When they cannot stabilize the segments, the vertebral ligaments are then forced to do this alone. They eventually become lax and subsequently cause pain. This is probably why back pain so commonly occurs several years after this operation. If the muscles and ligaments cannot stabilize the joints in the lower back, the vertebrae loosen and eventually rub together and crack, causing excessive bone growth in order to stabilize the joint. The stabilization results in spondylosis, or arthritis of the lumbar spine. Often the person then succumbs to another operation for the arthritis that formed as a result of the first operation. Unfortunately for the patient, the second operation is not a panacea of pain relief either. A simpler approach is Prolotherapy to correct the underlying ligament laxity which was causing the pain in the first place. This sequence of events is also applicable to other areas of the body. **(Figure 7-4)**

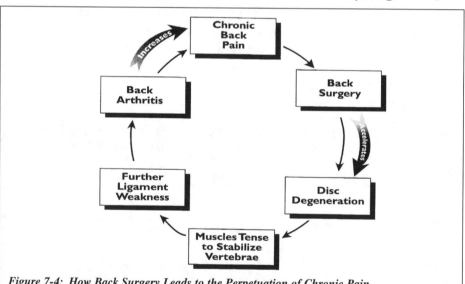

Figure 7-4: How Back Surgery Leads to the Perpetuation of Chronic Pain
Back surgery, by removing important tissue, puts greater strain on remaining tissues, which eventually weaken and become a source of chronic pain.

2. DISCECTOMY

Discectomy, another common back surgery, follows the same degenerative sequence as a laminectomy. Once the disc material is surgically removed, stress is added to the segments above and below the removed disc segment. These segments may eventually degenerate and become a cause of chronic pain. In a study by John Maynard, M.D., 10 percent of people after disc operation reherniated the same disc at a later date. Four years after surgery, 38 percent of the patients still had persistent pain in the back and 23 percent had persistent pain in the lower limbs.[13]

3. LUMBAR SPINAL FUSION

Lumbar spinal fusion operations fuse together several segments of the vertebrae. Such an operation is commonly performed for spondylolisthesis, a condition where one vertebral segment slips forward on another. **(See Figure 7-3.)** This causes back pain, especially when bending. By definition, spinal fusion causes permanent bonding or fusing of several vertebral segments. Mobility is decreased, causing increased stress on the areas above and below the fused segment. Over time, this stress may create weakened ligaments. The weakened ligaments lead to a degenerated disc which eventually leads to a degenerated spine resulting in a painfully stiff back.

Prolotherapy is a much safer and effective alternative to a laminectomy, a discectomy, or a lumbar spinal fusion. Prolotherapy initiates the repair process of the loose ligaments in spondylolisthesis and degenerated and herniated discs. For these reasons, Prolotherapy should be performed before a patient considers a surgical procedure to alleviate pain.

In her article, published in the *Journal of the American Medical Association* in 1992, "Patient Outcomes After Lumbar Spinal Fusions," Judith A. Turner, Ph.D., noted that there has never been a randomized or double-blind study comparing lumbar spinal fusion with any other technique. In some cases, only 16 percent of the people experienced satisfactory results after the operation. On average, 14 percent of the people experience incomplete healing of the surgical site. The most frequent symptom persisting after the operation is low back pain, which is often the reason for the operation in the first place. Turner concluded her article by saying that the wide variability in reported success rates is bothersome and should be carefully considered by patients and their physicians when contemplating this procedure.[14]

PROLOTHERAPY AFTER BACK SURGERY

Many people only become aware of Prolotherapy after they have undergone a surgical procedure for back pain. Although the pain may not be as severe as it was before the surgery, most people continue to experience significant back pain after surgery. Why? The back surgery involved removing supporting structure(s) such as a lamina, facet, or disc thus weakening surrounding segments.

Prolotherapy injections to the weakened segments in the lumbar vertebrae often result in definitive pain relief in post-surgery pain syndromes. Back pain is commonly due to several factors and surgery may have eliminated only one. It is possible, for example, to have back pain from a lumbar herniated disc and a sacroiliac joint problem. Surgery may address the herniated disc problem but not the sacroiliac problem. In this example, Prolotherapy injections to the sacroiliac joint would cure the chronic pain problem. **(Figure 7-5)**

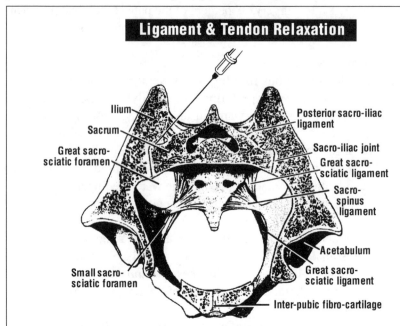

Ligament & Tendon Relaxation

Ilium

Sacrum

Great sacro-sciatic foramen

Posterior sacro-iliac ligament

Sacro-iliac joint

Great sacro-sciatic ligament

Sacro-spinus ligament

Acetabulum

Great sacro-sciatic ligament

Small sacro-sciatic foramen

Inter-pubic fibro-cartilage

Figure 7-5: Prolotherapy of the Sacroiliac Joint
Transverse section through sacroiliac joints with needle in position of full insertion to joint margin of posterior sacroiliac ligament.

Unfortunately it is common for a person to have lumbar spine surgery for a "sciatica" complaint diagnosed from an "abnormality" on an MRI scan. The "sciatica" complaint was a simple ligament problem in the sacroiliac joint and the MRI scan finding was not clinically relevant—it had nothing to do with the pain problem. For the majority of people who experience pain radiating down the leg, even in cases where numbness is present, the cause of the problem is not a pinched nerve but sacroiliac ligament weakness.

Ligament laxity in the sacroiliac joint is the number one reason for "sciatica" or pain radiating down the side of the leg, and is one of the most common reasons for chronic low back pain.[15] This can easily be confirmed by stretching these ligaments and producing a positive "jump sign." Ligament weakness can cause leg numbness. Most people sense pain when they have ligament weakness, but some people experience a sensation of numbness. Doctors typically believe nerve injury is the only reason for numbness, a reason so many people believe they have a sciatic nerve problem. In reality it is a sacroiliac ligament problem. The referral patterns of the sciatic nerve and the sacroiliac ligaments are similar. **(See Figures 2-2 to 2-5.)** In this scenario, it is unfortunate that thousands of dollars were spent on surgery and post-operative care. Had Prolotherapy treatments been performed on the pain-producing structure, this could have been avoided.

DIAGNOSIS OF ARACHNOIDITIS

Arachnoiditis is typically diagnosed in someone who has undergone back surgery and still suffers severe back pain that radiates down the legs and often to the feet. The pain has a persistent burning, stinging, or aching quality.[16] The diagnosis is occasionally made when similar symptoms are felt in the neck, arms, or the mid back with radiation into the chest. This pain is typically unresponsive to pain medications and muscle relaxants.

The term arachnoiditis signifies an inflammation of the arachnoid membrane which covers the spinal cord. The diagnosis of arachnoiditis is generally inaccurate because no signs of inflammation such as redness, fever, or an elevated sed rate (blood test that identifies inflammation) are seen in these patients. All that is seen is scar tissue on the MRI.

Arachnoiditis is another condition that is typically diagnosed by the large metal box with a magnet in it. For the patient who succumbed to surgery, only to be left with continued or worsened leg pains, repeated MRI and CAT scans are done. Eventually one of these scans will show some scar tissue. The physician will then inform the patient that the mysterious cause of the pain has been found, "You have arachnoiditis. Scar tissue is pinching the nerves."

It is common for someone with severe burning pains in the legs to receive a diagnostic study such as an MRI or CAT scan of the lower back. These tests are performed because they are supposed to reveal the source of the problem to the physician. The problem with this logic is that the MRI or CAT scan is designed to reveal density and configuration of structures, not diagnose conditions. Physicians are supposed to diagnose but unfortunately for many people with chronic pain, physicians have left the diagnosing to a large metal box with a magnet in it.

The patient in the above scenario is at first ecstatic because "the cause" of the pain has been found. The patient's jubilation is short-lived when the physician tells the patient that arachnoiditis is not curable, but the pain can be "controlled." Imagine having surgery for back and leg pain and coming out of the surgery with the same back and leg pain. The doctor then says the pain is due to scar tissue pinching on the nerves. How did the scar tissue get there? The answer is from the surgery of course.

The problem with this diagnosis is that the scar tissue was not present before the surgery, but the back and leg pains were. So what explains the back and leg pain that occurred before surgery? Answer that one and you will have the answer to why the person suffers from back and leg pain after surgery.

A more logical conclusion is that the surgery did not address the cause of the back and leg pain. Furthermore, the scar tissue seen on x-ray most likely has nothing to do with the current pain complaints of the patient. The number one cause of low back pain radiating into the legs is sacroiliac ligament laxity. Shooting pain down the leg is commonly due to ligament weakness in the lower back, including the sacroiliac, iliolumbar, sacrospinous, sacrotuberous, and hip joint ligaments. **(See Figures 2-2 and 2-5.)**

The person in the above scenario needed a Prolotherapist to relieve the pain, not a surgeon. Anyone carrying the diagnosis of arachnoiditis needs the immediate attention of a Prolotherapist before succumbing to epidural steroid injections, more surgeries, spinal cord stimulator implantation, or other invasive treatments which are only marginally helpful.[17, 18]

Arachnoiditis has been described as occurring after invasive treatments in and around the spinal column such as neck or back surgery, cortisone injections, spinal anesthetics, or myelography (a technique whereby dye is injected around the spinal cord to visualize the nerves).[19] The question is what percentage of people will develop a scar as evidenced on x-ray after back surgery? If you said 100 percent, you are correct. Each time a person undergoes surgery, a scar will develop. It is that simple.

Many people with the diagnosis of arachnoiditis have a repeat surgery to remove the scar tissue that is pinching on the nerves. Unfortunately, the results after a second surgery are dismal when it comes to permanent pain relief.

RESEARCH STUDY

A study consisting of 36 patients with arachnoiditis noted that each patient averaged three previous myelograms and three back surgeries.[21] They endured three pokes in the back for the myelogram and three knife treatments. Don't you think your x-ray would show scar tissue after all of that?! In this study, 88 percent of the patients were diagnosed with arachnoiditis by x-ray and the other 12 percent by surgery. Do you see a problem? What about a patient history? What about the thumb? A few pokes on the sacroiliac joint eliciting a positive "jump sign" and the cause of the pain would have been accurately identified.

Often people with the diagnosis of "arachnoiditis" experience significant difficulties in walking or holding down a job. The most startling result observed from the study was that the average life span was shortened by 12 years. Anyone who has had back surgery with recurrent pain should be evaluated for another cause of the pain besides arachnoiditis. Since scar tissue occurs 100 percent of the time after surgery, an MRI showing scar tissue should not be used to make a diagnosis. People who carry this diagnosis usually have the history of repeated tests and invasive procedures with the end result being a life expectancy shortened by 12 years.

Prolotherapy to the weakened structures such as the sacroiliac ligaments causing the pain will cure the condition and alleviate the pain. Once the weakened structure in the back becomes strong, the pain stops. Once the pain stops, the CAT and MRI scans and subsequent surgeries also stop. Consequently, many people with arachnoiditis are choosing to Prolo their pain away.

MID-UPPER BACK PAIN

James Cade, M.D., in Hattiesburg, Mississippi, described the following case to us: "W.M., a 34-year-old with severe mid-upper back pain between the shoulder blades, found no relief despite chronic use of Vicodin pain pills. The MRI, regular x-ray, and bone scan of W.M.'s thoracic spine showed no abnormalities. W.M. was offered surgery, costing $28,000, with little hope of success. I palpated the costovertebral ligaments and reproduced his pain. He agreed to the Prolotherapy injections and was on the way to healing his chronic pain."

This case illustrates many important points concerning routine chronic pain management. It is common for people to be offered surgery because nothing else has helped. Surgery should never be considered as routine as slicing a ham sandwich. Surgery involves someone cutting, slicing, grinding, tearing, and pulling out your body parts while you're asleep. It is our contention that if people were shown a video of the surgery prior to the operation, few would consent. No one should have surgery "just to try it." Surgery should only be performed for chronic pain management in the most extreme circumstances and only if all other conservative treatments have not been successful.

Most of the body's ligaments are not revealed on x-ray. The diagnosis of ligament injury is made by history and physical examination, not by x-ray. Dr. Cade was familiar with ligament injuries and their referral patterns and prevented W.M. from an unnecessary operation that in all likelihood would not have solved the problem. W.M. had ligament weakness at the rib-vertebrae junction, allowing his ribs to move too much which further stretched his costovertebral ligaments leading to more pain. Costovertebral ligament laxity often refers pain from the mid-upper back to the chest. **(See Figures 7-6, page 82.)** This is one of the causes for chronic chest discomfort.

Costovertebral ligament injuries are very slow to heal, or heal incompletely, because they are constantly under stress from the movement of the rib cage during breathing. The costovertebral junctions are prone to being injured any time the rib cage is jarred. This may occur from being hit in the chest, after receiving CPR, or from the effects of heart or thoracic surgery. During these types of surgeries the sternum is opened and the ribs are spread apart, commonly causing injury to the costovertebral junctions. In our opinion, chronic chest or upper-back discomfort after heart or lung surgery is almost always due to injury to the ligament support at the rib attachments in the thoracic spine or on the sternum. Prolotherapy is extremely effective at eliminating post-bypass chest or upper-back discomfort.

Prolotherapy, as in the case illustrated, is extremely effective at stabilizing vertebral segments and vertebral-rib segments. Costovertebral ligament laxity is a common cause of chronic mid-upper back or chest pain. This is why many people are choosing to Prolo their chronic mid-upper back and chest pain away.

Figure 7-6A: Physician Reproduces Pain at the Rib-Vertebrae Junction
Weakness at the rib-vertebrae (costovertebral) junction ligaments is a common source of mid-back pain.

Figure 7-6B: Referral Pain Pattern of the Rib-Sternal Junction
Rib-vertebrae (costovertebral) ligament weakness can cause pain to occur in the chest.

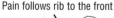
Pain follows rib to the front

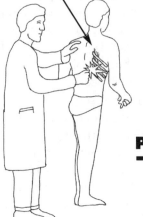

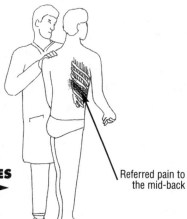
Referred pain in the front of the chest

PRODUCES

Pain follows rib to the back.

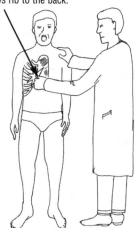

PRODUCES

Referred pain to the mid-back

Figure 7-6C: Physician Reproduces Pain at the Rib-Sternal Junction
Weakness at the rib-sternal (costochondral or sternocostal) ligament junction is a common source of chest pain.

Figure 7-6D: Referral Pain Pattern af the Rib-Vertebrae Junction
Rib-sternal (costochondral or sternocostal) ligament weakness can cause pain to occur in the side or mid-back region.

PAIN FROM SCOLIOSIS

Scoliosis is a lateral curvature of the spine of 11 degrees or more. An estimated 500,000 adults in the United States have scoliosis.[22] Scoliosis is usually discovered during adolescence and is called idiopathic scoliosis, a fancy term meaning the doctor has no idea what caused the scoliosis.

In common language, scoliosis means that the spine is crooked. The spine is held together by the same thing that holds all the bones together, ligaments. The patient often experiences pain at the site where the spine curves. At the apex of this curve, the ligaments are being stretched with the scoliosis, and localized ligament weakness is one of the etiological bases for it.

Traditional treatments for scoliosis, especially during adolescence, include observation, bracing, and surgery.[23, 24, 25] Observation of a crooked spine does not sound very helpful, bracing has been shown to decrease the progression of mild scoliosis, and surgery involves placing big rods in the back to stabilize the spine. Surgery is generally utilized for severe scoliosis when bracing has failed to stop the progression.

Again, every disease has a cause. Since scoliosis involves the spine moving in the wrong direction, treatment should be aimed at why this is occurring and correcting the problem. Ligament laxity is probably the main plausible explanation for the development of scoliosis and its pain. Prolotherapy treatments to strengthen the weakened ligaments can have potentially stabilizing and curative effects in scoliosis. If the scoliosis is progressing quickly, then bracing would be necessary in addition to Prolotherapy.

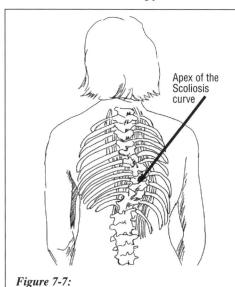

Figure 7-7:
Scoliosis of the Thoracic Vertebrae
Weakened ligaments at the apex of the curve cause pain in scoliosis.

Apex of the Scoliosis curve

Scoliosis pain has common patterns depending on where the scoliosis is located.[26] These pain patterns are easily reproduced by palpating the ligaments over the scoliotic segments of the spine. A positive "jump sign" will be elicited ensuring the diagnosis. The most common reason for pain with scoliosis is ligament weakness at the apex of the scoliosis curve. (**See Figure 7-7.**) Prolotherapy treatments over the entire scoliotic segment is effective at eliminating the pain of scoliosis. It has the added benefit of causing the ligaments to strengthen which will help stabilize the segment. For these reasons, Prolotherapy should be a part of comprehensive scoliosis management.

SUMMARY

In summary, the treatment that should be utilized in resistant cases of back pain is Prolotherapy. Prolotherapy eliminates chronic back pain in conditions such as degenerated discs, herniated discs, spondylolisthesis, post-surgery pain syndromes, arachnoiditis, and scoliosis. The most common cause of chronic low back pain and "sciatica" is laxity of the sacroiliac ligaments. Prolotherapy should be tried before any surgical procedure is performed for chronic back pain. Prolotherapy is an extremely effective treatment for chronic low back pain because it permanently strengthens the structures that are causing the pain. It is for this reason that many people are choosing to Prolo their chronic back pain away. ■

CHAPTER 8

Prolo All Your Degenerative Conditions Away!

CASE HISTORY

Helen called us crying on the phone. Both of her knees had given out, she was in terrible pain, and was unable to get out of the bed. Helen was in bad shape. When we saw her, Helen relayed to us that she recently underwent a knee arthroscopy. The orthopedist told her that her knees were shot. No cartilage or ligaments were left to hold everything together. She was told to just sit and wait until she could afford a knee replacement. Helen was financially strapped because she was unable to perform her job of cleaning houses due to the bad knees. The outlook did not look good for Helen. She was looking at facing the welfare system, unemployment, and trying to find a way to feed her family. All she could do was cry. Upon physical examination, the orthopedist was right, her knees were shot. There was no cartilage and very loose, weak ligaments.

We asked Helen how she got into this condition in the first place, being that she was only 37 years old. She explained that as a youngster she would entertain the other kids by bending her knees backward. She was apparently born with very loose ligaments.

Helen received her first Prolotherapy treatment to her knees that day. She needed more than the typical four or five treatments because of the severity of her case. Prolotherapy was a much better option for a 37 year-old than a knee replacement.

Immediately after the injections, Helen was able to stand up and stated that her knees already felt better. The little bit of anesthetic in the Prolotherapy solution, which was injected directly into the painful areas, provided immediate pain relief. Helen received nine Prolotherapy sessions over the next several months. After the second set of Prolotherapy injections she experienced enough pain relief to start scrubbing floors. She was instructed to wear kneepads while she worked and to stop entertaining the kids by bending the knees backwards. She has lived a wonderful four years without pain. Yes, her knees were shot, but she received new knees as evidenced by the amount of cartilage in her post-Prolotherapy x-rays. **(See Helen's actual x-rays, Figure 8-1.)** The best part is that her new knees came without a surgeon's knife, but by the gentle touch of a Prolotherapy syringe!

DEGENERATIVE JOINT DISEASE VERSUS AGING

Getting old has nothing to do with getting pain! Many people come in to our office, doubtful that anything could help them, resigning themselves to living with chronic pain because they are older. Hogwash! There is always a cause for chronic pain. The cause is not old age. This is exemplified when looking at the articular cartilage in the joints of an older person versus the joints of someone with

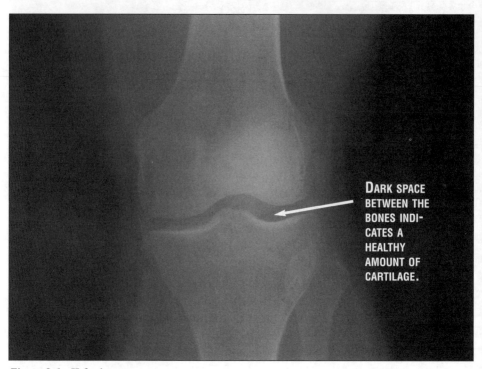

DARK SPACE BETWEEN THE BONES INDICATES A HEALTHY AMOUNT OF CARTILAGE.

Figure 8-1: Helen's x-ray
Prolotherapy stimulates the body to repair the painful area, including cartilage.

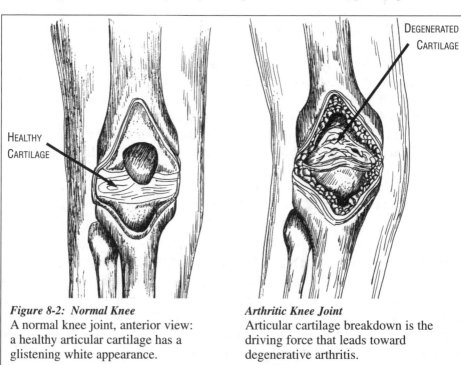

DEGENERATED CARTILAGE

HEALTHY CARTILAGE

Figure 8-2: Normal Knee
A normal knee joint, anterior view: a healthy articular cartilage has a glistening white appearance.

Arthritic Knee Joint
Articular cartilage breakdown is the driving force that leads toward degenerative arthritis.

osteoarthritis (degenerative arthritis) at any age. The joints look totally and completely different! The articular cartilage of the aging person looks nothing like the articular cartilage of a patient with arthritis. (**See Figure 8-2.**)

Pain is the body's signal that something is wrong, weakened, or injured. The most commonly injured tissues in the chronic pain sufferer are the ligaments that stabilize the joints. It is the laxity or weakness in these tissues that produces most degenerative joint disease. This is why Helen, even at age 37, had severe degeneration in her knees.

The bones in a joint such as the knee are no longer held in a stable position following an injury to the ligaments. This leads to instability in the knee with eventual crunching in the joint. Crunching in a joint is a sure sign that the joint-stabilizing structures are in a weakened state. A person who receives Prolotherapy at this point can stop this whole downward spiral. If the joint instability is not treated, the degeneration in the joint will continue. Eventually this will lead to articular cartilage breakdown. Even at this point, Prolotherapy, in conjunction with nutritional remedies can help regenerate the injured tissue. If left untreated, all of the articular cartilage will erode and the person will be left with a joint that is stiff and painful. The orthopedist will call the condition "bone on bone." Prolotherapy can still be tried for "bone on bone" but it is not as successful as when the degenerative process is only mild to moderate. These patients typically experience some pain relief, but not complete relief. To some people, partial pain relief is worth it.

Degenerative joint conditions almost always start because of a soft tissue injury to the joint. Generally this is an injury to the ligaments, the stabilizing structures of the joint. When the ligaments are stretched and weakened, the other structures in the joint must perform functions that they were not designed to do. Eventually these structures become fatigued and cartilage begins to break down.

COMMON DEGENERATIVE CONDITIONS TREATED SUCCESSFULLY WITH PROLOTHERAPY

AREA	CONDITION
KNEE	Osteoarthritis, Chondromalacia Patellae
HIP	Osteoarthritis, Hip Ligament Sprain
LOWER BACK	Degenerated Disc, Herniated Disc
NECK	Degenerated Disc, Herniated Disc
SHOULDER	Osteoarthritis, Rotator Cuff Tendonitis
ANKLE/FEET	Ankle Ligament Sprains, Plantar Fasciitis
HANDS/FINGERS	Osteoarthritis, Ligament Sprains

Figure 8-3

This process is commonly experienced in the hip and knee joints. This is the reason why over 120,000 hip replacements and 95,000 knee replacements are performed each year in the United States alone.[1,2]

WHAT IS OSTEOARTHRITIS?

Osteoarthritis is the most common form of arthritis affecting many of the population over the age of fifty. It is also called "degenerative joint disease" because osteoarthritis involves the deterioration of the articular cartilage that lines the joints and related changes in adjacent bone and joint margins. This deterioration occurs because the supporting structures of the joints, primarily the ligaments, become injured. The joint then becomes unstable, loose, and moves excessively. The crunching noises in the joints commonly seen with this condition occur because the bones start hitting together. An overgrowth of bone forms at the areas where the bones are hitting (generally at the joint margins). This overgrowth of bone along with the articular cartilage damage is called osteoarthritis or degenerative joint disease (DJD).

DJD most frequently occurs in the weight-bearing articulations of the spine, hips, and knees, and the distal interphalangeal joints of the hands. Symptoms of DJD usually include brief joint stiffness upon awakening, joint pain or tenderness following usage, and are associated with the typical characteristic findings on x-ray. The most common DJD conditions treated with Prolotherapy are exhibited in **Figure 8-3**.

The common thinking about DJD is that it occurs due to wear and tear on the joints and is inevitable as you age. Nothing could be farther from the truth! Its root cause is almost always **injury** to the soft tissue supporting structures of the joint. The process of developing DJD begins with ligament weakness. More than twelve studies were done that showed that DJD does not occur as a result of wear and tear. The studies included 1597 individuals, with an average age of fifty-three years, who ran an average of thirty-three miles per week for approximately sixteen years. There was no evidence of an increased occurrence of DJD in these people.[3] Prolotherapy also confirms this theory because the pain and disability from DJD are resolved when the ligamentous structures around the joint are treated with Prolotherapy. The process of arthritis and DJD formation is **halted** with Prolotherapy by strengthening the joints' supporting structures. The arthritic process is then completely stopped!

Unfortunately, most people continue to perpetuate the arthritic/DJD process by using the RICE protocol. Anti-inflammatory medications, cortisone shots, arthroscopy, and the various surgeries offered to people (all part of the RICE protocol) with degenerative joint disease all contribute to the downward spiral in the development of arthritis/DJD. All of these treatments help destroy the articular cartilage, which is the very structure that prevents us from getting arthritis and DJD. It will be your choice; choose arthritis for your future or choose Prolotherapy.

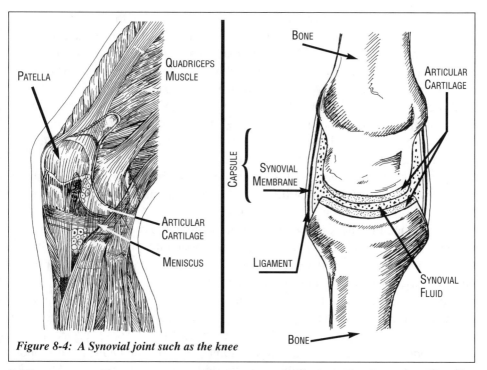

Figure 8-4: A Synovial joint such as the knee

WHAT IS ARTICULAR CARTILAGE? IS IT IN CRISIS?

Most of the joints in the body are synovial joints. These are movable, highly versatile, lubricated joints. Synovial joints are able to provide normal pain-free movement because of the unique properties of the articular cartilage. The articular cartilage of the synovial joint covers and protects the ends of the bones. Ligaments help provide stability to the joint. A fibrous capsule encloses the structure for protection. Muscles around the joint contract to produce movement. The knee is the largest synovial joint. We will use the knee and hip joints as the primary examples in our discussion on "the cartilage crisis."

Let us examine the knee in more detail. In **Figure 8-4,** at the top of the knee are the massive quadriceps muscles that cause the knee to extend. The hamstring muscles are at the back of the knee and cause it to flex. The knee joint contains a synovial membrane, which is tissue that lines the non-contact surfaces within the joint capsule. This tissue secretes lubricating synovial fluid, which nourishes all the tissues inside the joint capsule. The stabilizing structures of the knee during movement are the cruciate ligaments (internal joint ligaments) and the collateral ligaments (external joint ligaments). The menisci, which are unique to the knee and the wrist, are pads of fibrous cartilage, which help the weight-bearing bones absorb shock. The ends of the tibia, femur, and patellar bones of the knee joint are covered by articular cartilage. This is the structure that is in crisis.

Articular cartilage plays a vital role in the function of the musculoskeletal system by allowing almost frictionless motion to occur between the surfaces of two bones.[4] Furthermore, articular cartilage distributes the load of the joint articulation over a larger contact area, thereby minimizing the contact stresses, and dissipating the energy force associated with the load.[5] These properties allow the potential for articular cartilage to remain healthy and fully functional throughout decades of life despite the very slow turnover rate of its collagen matrix.

Articular cartilage is normally glassy, white, and very homogeneous in its structure. It is an avascular tissue (no blood vessels), devoid of nerves and lymphatic vessels, and contains just a few cells (chondrocytes) that are embedded in a sea of collagen. Specialized protein structures called proteoglycans, water, and collagen make up the structure. It is the chemical nature and arrangement of these structures that gives articular cartilage its resilience, durability, strength, and efficient weight-bearing and gliding properties.[6]

The average thickness of the articular cartilage in the knee is two to four millimeters. The thickest cartilage of the knee appears on the patella at five millimeters or more.[7] There is no evidence to suggest that the thickness of articular cartilage decreases with age in a healthy individual.[8]

Although the surface of articular cartilage appears smooth on gross examination under electron microscopy, there are depressions and undulations. There are actually about 430 depressions per millimeter of cartilage.[9] These surface irregularities appear to play an important role in joint lubrication and nutritional support by trapping the nutrient-rich, thick synovial fluid.

The cells (chondrocytes) of articular cartilage are responsible for the synthesis of both the collagen and proteoglycans that make up the cartilage. The chondrocytes have the ability to synthesize all the various components of the specialized proteins that make up the proteoglycans.[10]

The ability of these chondrocytes to replicate is really the key question when considering the potential of cartilage to proliferate or repair itself. It has been shown in studies on adult human cartilage that no decrease in cell count occurs with age.[11] This fact only suggests that chondrocytes have the ability to proliferate and repair.

Upon injury, such as mild compression,[12] osteoarthritis,[13] or lacerative injury, the chondrocytes can revert back to a "chondroblastic" state. This is a condition where the chondrocytes are capable of mitotic division, indicative of growth and proliferation.[14] The notion of damaged cartilage having no regenerative properties is responsible for many people being subjected to arthroscopies with subsequent joint replacements. This falsehood occurred because healthy cartilage cells have very little, if any, mitotic activity, thus very little or no ability to proliferate.[15] The fact that healthy cartilage cells (chondrocytes) have no ability to proliferate and repair was discovered in the early 1960's. The first total hip replacement surgery occurred at the same time. A short time later the arthroscope was invented. These occurrences led to the massive proliferation of orthopedic surgery and surgeons throughout the country. Since articular cartilage reportedly had no ability to heal, then removal of any damaged articular cartilage was justified.

CARTILAGE REGENERATION

Much of the research on articular cartilage regeneration was done in the 1980's and 1990's. Not until the early 1980's did Dr. H.J. Mankin discover that the chondrocytes' reaction to injury was to change into a more immature cell called a chondroblast. This type of cell, interestingly enough, is capable of cell proliferation, growth, and healing.[16] His research is so well-accepted that two of his papers on this subject were published in one of the most prestigious medical journals in the world, *The New England Journal of Medicine.*[17, 18] The actual cells that make collagen (chondrocytes) and the other components of articular cartilage gain the ability to replicate, proliferate, and generate new cartilage upon injury. This key fact is vital to understanding the power of Prolotherapy to proliferate cartilage growth.

Prolotherapy involves the injection of various substances, including hypertonic dextrose, sodium morrhuate (an extract of cod liver oil), various minerals, Sarapin (an extract of the pitcher plant), and various other substances. Many of these substances act by causing a mild irritation at the site of the injection. It is believed that this irritation acts in the same mechanism as above for cartilage formation by inducing the chondrocytes to change to the chondroblastic stage of development. Prolotherapy regenerates cartilage most likely by inducing mature chondrocytes to a chondroblastic state capable of proliferation and repair. This fact is supported by the numerous patients with "no cartilage" set for hip/knee replacements who never needed them after receiving Prolotherapy. It is also supported by the numerous patients like Helen who were told that arthroscopy revealed that their cartilage was completely gone, yet chose to try Prolotherapy, only to live long, happy, productive lives. Helen, as you recall, was even able to scrub floors on her knees again. Not that we all cherish doing that task. There is no other explanation for the radical transformation of Helen's cartilage from deterioration to a healthy state—Prolotherapy!

Prolotherapy can help regenerate articular cartilage. This is a good thing. How, on the other hand, did the articular cartilage of all the joints become so deteriorated? How does this happen? It happens because people listen to their doctors.

THE MIGHTY MENISCUS—ART'S BEST FRIEND

Articular cartilage has very few friends. Everything is working against him. He has to handle hundreds of pounds with each step and he gets fed scraps from the synovial fluid. Not a job anyone of us would want. He has a best friend however, the mighty meniscus ("Minny" for short.)

The menisci are C-shaped disks of fibrocartilage interposed between the condyles of the femur and tibia. They are composed of about 75 percent collagen, 8 to 13 percent protein, and the rest extracellular matrix component.[19] Type I collagen makes up about 90 percent of the total collagen.[20] This is the same type of collagen that makes up ligaments and tendons. **(See Figure 8-5.)**

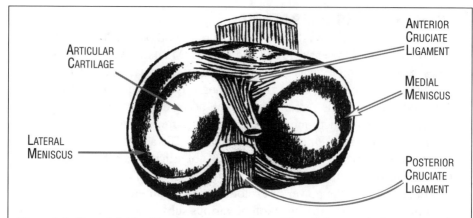

ARTICULAR
CARTILAGE

ANTERIOR
CRUCIATE
LIGAMENT

MEDIAL
MENISCUS

LATERAL
MENISCUS

POSTERIOR
CRUCIATE
LIGAMENT

Figure 8-5: Knee joint looking from the top, down. The mighty menisci are responsible for shock absorption and lubrication.

The size of the meniscus relative to its corresponding tibial plateau remains remarkably constant throughout development and into adulthood. On the average, the medial meniscus covers about 64 percent of the medial tibial plateau, while the lateral meniscus covers about 84 percent of the lateral tibial plateau.[21] The medial meniscus is larger in diameter than the lateral meniscus. It has an average width of 10 millimeters, and is 3 to 5 millimeters thick. The lateral meniscus has a thickness of 3 to 5 millimeters, with an average width of 12 to 13 millimeters.[22]

The mighty menisci are responsible for load transmission, shock absorption, lubrication, and improvement of stability of the knees. Most studies indicate that the menisci transmit about 50 percent of the load at the knee, while the remaining 50 percent is borne directly by the articular cartilage and surfaces.[23, 24] The menisci therefore protect the articular cartilage from high concentrations of stress by increasing the contact area on the femur and tibia bones. Removing the menisci is probably one of the worse possible scenarios for the articular cartilage because it would decrease the contact area onto the bones and would significantly increase the forces onto the articular cartilage itself. It would only make sense that removing the menisci should be a last resort for the athlete, as it will only make the problem worse in the long run.

Essentially every study shows that articular cartilage pressures escalate when the menisci are removed. Ahmed and Burke showed a 40 percent increase in the contact stress while Baratz and associates found a 235 percent increase in articular cartilage contact force following total meniscectomy.[25, 26] If that is not bad enough, other researchers found 450 to 700 percent increases in articular cartilage pressure. A reasonable average estimate taken from the available literature indicates that total meniscectomy results in a two- to three-fold (200-300 percent) increase in contact stresses.[27, 28, 29]

Removal of the menisci will produce one end result: a degenerated knee sometime in the future. The time is usually sooner rather than later. Following partial

College graduation from the University of Illinois in Champaign-Urbana.

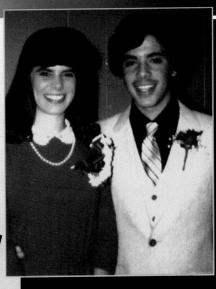

One of our first dates in 1980.

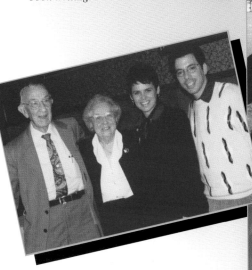

Squeaky Hauser takes a break from the book writing.

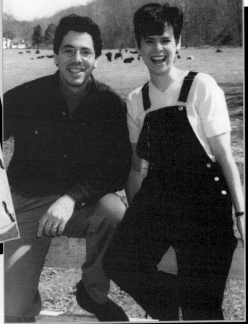

The Hemwalls and the Hausers— the history and the future of Prolotherapy.

Down on the farm, in Thebes, IL.

CARING MEDICAL AND REHABILITATION SERVICES

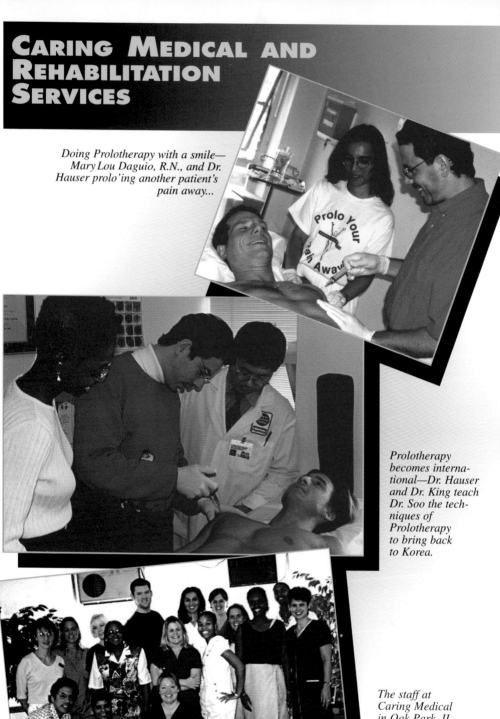

Doing Prolotherapy with a smile— Mary Lou Daguio, R.N., and Dr. Hauser prolo'ing another patient's pain away...

Prolotherapy becomes international—Dr. Hauser and Dr. King teach Dr. Soo the techniques of Prolotherapy to bring back to Korea.

The staff at Caring Medical in Oak Park, IL.

"The care of the patient begins with Caring."

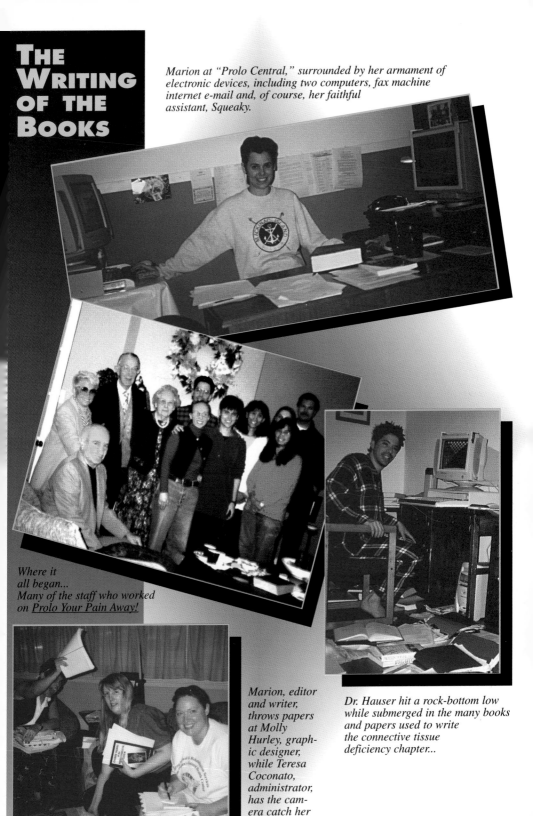

THE WRITING OF THE BOOKS

Marion at "Prolo Central," surrounded by her armament of electronic devices, including two computers, fax machine internet e-mail and, of course, her faithful assistant, Squeaky.

Where it all began...
Many of the staff who worked on Prolo Your Pain Away!

Marion, editor and writer, throws papers at Molly Hurley, graphic designer, while Teresa Coconato, administrator, has the camera catch her "good side."

Dr. Hauser hit a rock-bottom low while submerged in the many books and papers used to write the connective tissue deficiency chapter...

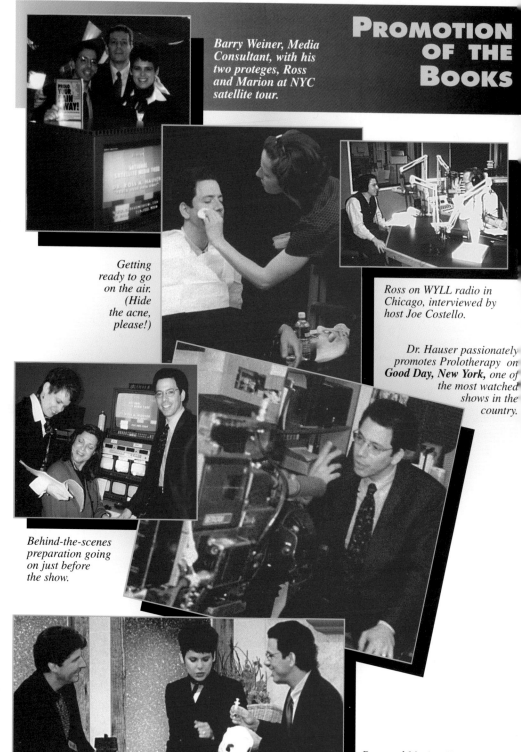

PROMOTION OF THE BOOKS

Barry Weiner, Media Consultant, with his two proteges, Ross and Marion at NYC satellite tour.

Getting ready to go on the air. (Hide the acne, please!)

Ross on WYLL radio in Chicago, interviewed by host Joe Costello.

*Dr. Hauser passionately promotes Prolotherapy on **Good Day, New York,** one of the most watched shows in the country.*

Behind-the-scenes preparation going on just before the show.

Ross and Marion Hauser discuss the technique of Prolotherapy with national radio and T.V. host Doug Kaufmann.

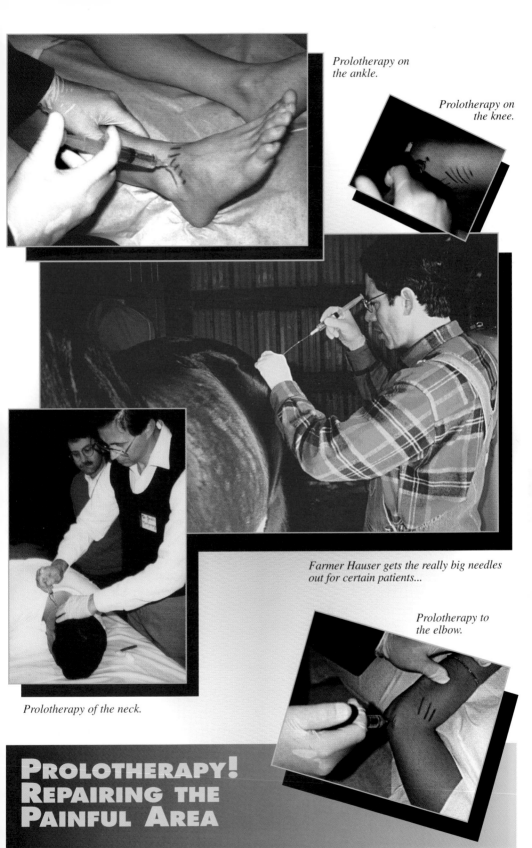

Prolotherapy on the ankle.

Prolotherapy on the knee.

Farmer Hauser gets the really big needles out for certain patients...

Prolotherapy to the elbow.

Prolotherapy of the neck.

PROLOTHERAPY!
REPAIRING THE
PAINFUL AREA

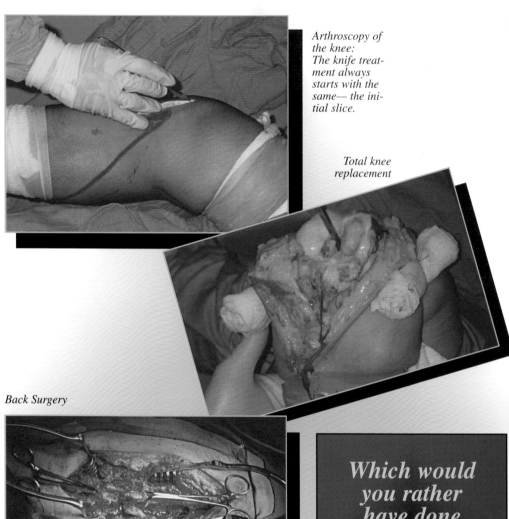

Arthroscopy of the knee: The knife treatment always starts with the same— the initial slice.

Total knee replacement

Back Surgery

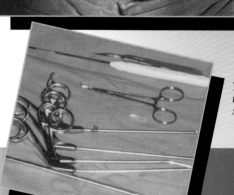

The Assault: tools of surgery.

Which would you rather have done to relieve your pain?

Surgery or Prolotherapy?

ALTERNATIVES TO PROLOTHERAPY: ARTHROSCOPY AND SURGERY

HACKETT-HEMWALL-HAUSER LIGAMENT REFERRAL PATTERNS

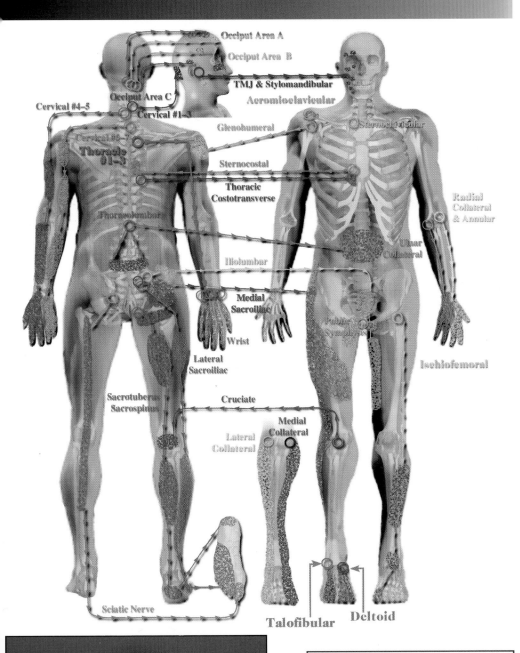

Occiput Area A
Occiput Area B
Occiput Area C
TMJ & Stylomandibular
Acromioclavicular
Cervical #4–5
Cervical #1–3
Sternoclavicular
Glenohumeral
Cervical #6
Thoracic #1–3
Sternocostal
Thoracic Costotransverse
Thoracolumbar
Radial Collateral & Annular
Ulnar Collateral
Iliolumbar
Medial Sacroiliac
Pubic Symphysis
Wrist
Ischiofemoral
Lateral Sacroiliac
Sacrotuberus Sacrospinus
Cruciate
Medial Collateral
Lateral Collateral
Sciatic Nerve
Talofibular
Deltoid

Ligament laxity can cause localized pain as well as refer to distant sites.

 = Ligament attachment sites
 = Ligament pain referral pattern
 = Ligament pain referral area

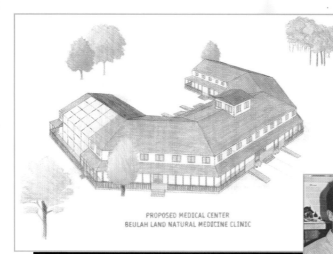

Artist's rendering of the future site of the Beulah Land Natural Medicine Clinic.

PROPOSED MEDICAL CENTER
BEULAH LAND NATURAL MEDICINE CLINIC

BEULAH LAND MINISTRIES

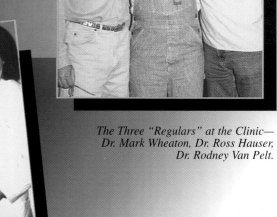

Dr. Rodney Van Pelt and Brodie Hackney at the Beulah Land missionary clinic.

The Three "Regulars" at the Clinic— Dr. Mark Wheaton, Dr. Ross Hauser, Dr. Rodney Van Pelt.

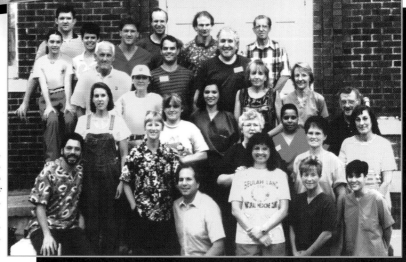

Many of the volunteers outside the First Baptist Church of Thebes, where the Beulah Land missionary clinic is held four times per year.

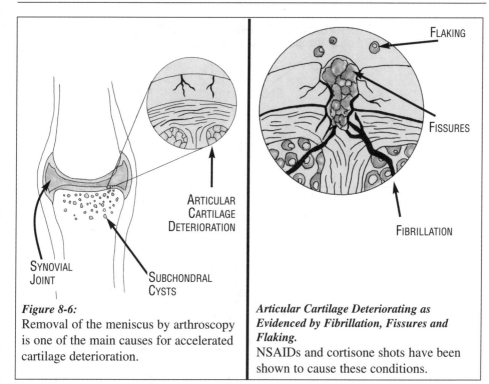

Figure 8-6:
Removal of the meniscus by arthroscopy is one of the main causes for accelerated cartilage deterioration.

Articular Cartilage Deteriorating as Evidenced by Fibrillation, Fissures and Flaking.
NSAIDs and cortisone shots have been shown to cause these conditions.

or total meniscectomy, articular degenerative changes have been described, including the formation of osteophytic ridges, generalized flattening of the femoral articular surface, and narrowing of the joint space. Roughening and degeneration of the articular cartilage is seen and seems to be proportional to the size of the segment removed. Degenerative changes appear first in the tibiofemoral contact areas, with those areas formerly covered by the meniscus involved later.[30, 31]

Once the menisci are removed, aggressive proliferative arthritis is inevitable. It occurs early in 40 percent of the people, but is essentially guaranteed long-term.[32, 33, 34] This sad fact needs serious consideration when an arthroscopy is proposed. Arthroscopic partial meniscectomy is an extremely common procedure performed in athletes. Besides the proliferative arthritis that results, a concomitant decrease in the ability to play athletics follows. Athletes, listen! Let no one, especially someone in a white coat with an arthroscope, do anything to your menisci. The health of your articular cartilage depends upon it! The pathogenesis of arthritis following meniscectomy is shown in **Figure 8-6.**

Meniscal removal leads to increased forces on the articular cartilage. This may produce articular cartilage breakdown, which leads to thinning of the articular cartilage. As a result of this, increased pressure on the underlying tibia bone is observed, which leads to more pressure on the ligaments. Ligament tears and chronic pain often result, which further weakens the joint. In response to this weakness, the joint overgrows bone, which is called arthritis.

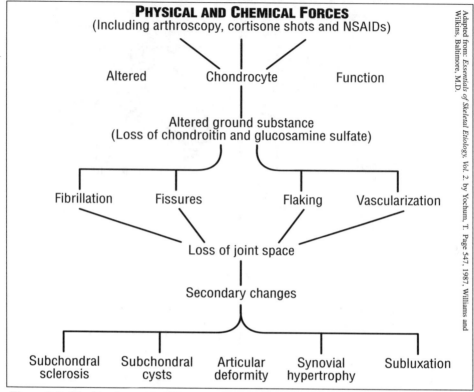

Adapted from: *Essentials of Skeletal Etiology*, Vol. 2. by Yochum, T. Page 547, 1987. Williams and Wilkins, Baltimore, M.D.

Figure 8-7: The Development of Degenerative Joint Disease

The process can be accelerated by arthroscopy, cortisone shots, and NSAIDs, the primary "tools" of most traditional pain doctors.

ARTHROSCOPY: THE QUICKEST WAY TO ARTHRITIS

All athletes need to remember this fact: There is a high likelihood that you will develop aggressive arthritis in the future if an arthroscope enters your knee joints. In fact, because arthroscopy is no longer reserved for athletes, **everyone** should beware. This does not apply to complete ligament tears. These may actually need surgical repair for an athlete to regain function. For all the other conditions, any tissue removal inside the knee will most likely give you an increased chance of a future filled with arthritis and the accompanying pain and a lessened ability to play sports or perform daily activities. A well-accepted schemata on the development of arthritis is shown in **Figure 8-7.**

Arthritis begins immediately after chondrocyte function is altered. This leads to altered production of ground substance or proteoglycans. Because the articular cartilage is now in a weakened state, breakdown begins. Orthopedists have fancy terms for this breakdown such as fibrillation, fissures, flaking, and vascularization. When they use these terms it just means your cartilage is going to pot. When articular cartilage thins this shows on x-ray as a loss of joint space. This causes a transmission of pressures that are too high for the bones to handle. The tibial bone in the knee, for example, will attempt to harden by sclerosis, forming cysts. The bone itself will actually overgrow to stabilize the area. This is why arthritic joints are called articular deformity, which is actually bone overgrowth.

Arthritis is not a pleasant thing to have. Anyone with a grandparent in pain from arthritis knows that this is no way to spend retirement. Remember any physical or chemical force that alters chondrocyte function and thus proteoglycan formation will have a tremendous impact on the cartilage crisis.

The effect on the patient who receives an arthroscopy is to provide a direct assault to the tissues. It is very rare for an orthopedist to just look into a joint. Tissue is shaved and cut because the physician truly believes that this helps the person. Even if the area is fibrillated or has frayed edges, how could removing the tissue possibly help the individual? It does nothing to help repair the area. Clinical experience indicates that arthroscopic shaving or abrasion of fibrillated and irregular cartilage may relieve symptoms temporarily, but long-term it can do nothing but aid in the arthritic process. Many times the argument is made that the cartilage was smoothed by arthroscopy. This now smoother cartilage (because the fibrillations and frayed edges were shaved) will allow a more normal glide of the bones. The research does not support this. Schmid and Schmid reported that shaving did not restore a smooth congruent articular surface and may have caused increased fibrillation and cell necrosis in and adjacent to the original defect.[35]

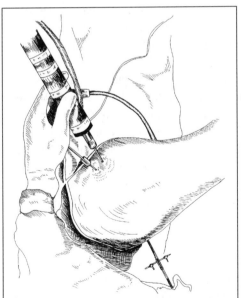

Figure 8-8: The Technique of Arthroscopy
The procedure generally involves the removal of structures with the end result being temporary pain relief—but long-term arthritis.

The best approach to help heal the injured area is Prolotherapy. At minimum an athlete should first try Prolotherapy because arthroscopy can always be done later. In over 12,000 patients treated with Prolotherapy by Dr. Gustav Hemwall and myself, only a rare patient has ever needed an arthroscopy referral. Knee conditions respond beautifully to Prolotherapy. This is because Prolotherapy stimulates the inflammatory process to heal the injured area.

PROLOTHERAPY VS. ARTHROSCOPY

Prolotherapy has many advantages over arthroscopy. It is, first of all, a much safer and conservative treatment. It works faster. The procedure does not

PROLOTHERAPY VERSUS ARTHROSCOPY

	PROLOTHERAPY	ARTHROSCOPY
STIMULATES REPAIR?	Yes	No
INCREASES COLLAGEN STRENGTH?	Yes	No
ARTHRITIS RISK?	Decreased	Increased
RETURN TO SPORT?	Quick	Slow
REHABILITATION TIME?	Short	Long
EXERCISE?	Encouraged	Cautious
COST?	Hundreds	Thousands
TIME INVOLVED IN PROCEDURE?	Minutes	Hours
INSTRUMENT USED?	Thin needle	Massive Scopes

Figure 8-9: Which would you rather have—Prolotherapy OR Arthroscopy?

take long to administer to the patient. The athlete is in and out of the doctor's office in less than an hour. Prolotherapy stimulates the body to heal the painful area. The new collagen tissue formed is actually stronger. It reduces the chance of long-term arthritis, whereas arthroscopy increases the chances for it. In many ways arthroscopy almost guarantees arthritis. Prolotherapy also increases the chances of athletes being able to play their sports for the rest of their lives. Arthroscopy significantly decreases those chances. Athletes may return to activity almost immediately after Prolotherapy. Athletes are encouraged to exercise while getting Prolotherapy, whereas after arthroscopy, athletes must often be very cautious and undergo extensive rehabilitation programs. The procedure itself is also much less invasive than putting massive scopes into the knee or shoulder. Arthroscopy requires the joint to be blown up with 100 millimeters of fluid to fit all the scopes into the knee or shoulder. **(See Figure 8-8.)**

Prolotherapy is easier on the pocket book than surgery. Prolotherapy usually costs between $200-300 per session. Arthroscopy costs several thousand dollars. Including rehabilitation the costs can be upwards of $10,000.

There are many other advantages to using Prolotherapy over arthroscopy with athletes or chronic pain patients. **(See Figure 8-9.)** The point is, the verdict is in! Say, "Nope to scope!"

RICE IS NOT ALWAYS NICE!

RICE stands for rest, ice, compression, and elevation. It generally involves resting or immobilizing the joint for some time because of an injury. Athletes are often taped, braced, casted, or told to rest because their injuries will not heal. Nothing could be worse for the articular cartilage throughout the joints of the body than this. The articular cartilage can only receive nourishment from the synovial fluid when it is pushed into the joint by weight bearing and loading. The cartilage has no blood supply of its own. Moving, exercising, and loading the joint will allow the nourishment to get into the articular cartilage and the waste products to get out. There is only one effect of RICE and immobilization on cartilage—it is not good.

It has been shown in basic animal research that in as little as six days of immobilizing a joint, pressure necrosis of the articular cartilage can occur with subsequent degenerative arthritis.[36] Another study showed that prolonged immobilization, as occurs with casting, can lead to degeneration of the articular cartilage even in noncontact areas secondary to the adhesion of synovial membrane to the joint surface, which would not happen if the joints were moved. Subsequent use of such immobilized joints also led to degenerative arthritis.[37]

As expected immobilization causes a fall in chondrocyte synthesis.[38] The chondrocytes cannot be nourished without movement, so their ability to make collagen and proteoglycans for the articular cartilage declines with immobility. Studies have confirmed that simple immobilization causes a thinning of articular cartilage and specifically, decrease in the glycosaminoglycan and chondroitin sulfate.[50, 51] Exercise, on the other hand, has a dramatic effect of increasing chondrocyte synthesis.[41] This would be expected since exercise enhances the ability of the chondrocytes to receive nutrients and eliminate waste.

Exercise has the following beneficial effects:

● Enhances the nutrition and metabolic activity of articular cartilage
● Stimulates pluripotential mesenchymal cells to differentiate into articular cartilage
● Accelerates healing of both articular cartilage and periarticular tissues, such as tendons and ligaments[42]

The above was all proven by the many studies done by Dr. Robert Salter at the University of Toronto. Dr. Robert Salter is the father of the theory that a limb must be continuously moved after an injury. He found that the healing rate was six times greater comparing movement and exercise with immobility in patients with articular cartilage defects.[43] Articular cartilage injuries which are rested have an over 50 percent chance of causing compromised range of motion of the limb at one year. Cartilage damaged limbs that are exercised had completely normal motion. Articular cartilage defects in rabbits that were immobilized caused 50 percent of them to get arthritis at one year. None had visible evidence of arthritis in the exercised group.[44]

Dr. Salter showed that 80 percent of articular cartilage fractures healed with exercise and movement, where none healed in the immobilized group. In an interesting study on infected joints, they showed that continuous passive motion of the joint had a striking and statistically significant protective effect on prevention of progressive degeneration of the articular cartilage when compared with the effects of immobilization.[45]

He felt the possible explanations for these findings were the following:

- Prevention of adhesions (scar tissue)
- Improvement of nutrition of the cartilage through increased diffusion of synovial fluid
- Enhancement of clearance of lysosomal enzymes and purulent exudate from the infected joints (removal of the bad stuff)
- Stimulation of living chondrocytes to synthesize the various components of the matrix

The mechanism by which exercise improved healing is not particularly clear. However, Dr. Salter did show by x-ray and clinical findings that the animals that received exercise did much better than the ones who were immobilized. This same statement could be said about Prolotherapy. We do not know the exact mechanism of action that Prolotherapy uses to help people heal. The positive results of patients speak for themselves.

Continuous passive motion exercise was also shown to heal or clear a hemarthrosis (blood in the joint) twice as fast as immobilized limbs.[46] This is significant for athletes who have massive bruising of a joint. The notion that the area must be iced and compressed to decrease swelling is outdated. Ice and compression will decrease swelling, but will compromise healing. Yes, there is a better way. The best way to resolve swelling is to use the MEAT treatment. This involves exercise and proteolytic enzymes, which help clean out the damaged tissue. **(See Chapter 5 for more on this topic.)** Exercise or passive motion by a physical therapist is tremendously effective at helping resolve the bleeding and edema but will also aid the healing process.

Dr. Salter summarized his first 18 years of basic research on the biologic concept of continuous passive motion (CPM) exercise with the following conclusions:

- CPM exercise is well tolerated
- CPM exercise has a significant stimulating effect on the healing of articular tissues, including cartilage, tendons, and ligaments
- CPM exercise prevents adhesions and joint stiffness
- CPM exercise does not interfere with the healing of incisions over the moving joint
- The time-honored principle that healing tissues must be put to rest is incorrect: indeed—it is this principle that must be put to rest rather than the healing soft tissues
- Regeneration of articular cartilage through neochondrogenesis both with and without periosteal grafts is possible under the influence of CPM exercise[47]

Dr. Salter wrote those words in the 1980's, yet there are still athletes around the world doing the RICE protocol today. Putting injured tissues to rest hurts the healing process. Animals continue their activities after an injury, therefore they heal well after an injury. Human beings need to do the same. It is time for a paradigm shift from the RICE to MEAT protocol to encourage healing of the soft tissue and cartilage injuries. Exercise is vital to this process.

Anti-inflame Your Cartilage Injury— and It Will Stay!

Again, the reason why arthritis forms in the first place is because an injured area did not heal. The pain of the initial injury may have been relieved, but the injured tissue remains injured, as manifested by decreased strength. Exercise alone does not cause arthritis. Only injury causes arthritis. In a study where dogs were exercised for one year carrying jackets weighing 130 percent of their body weight, all knee joints were inspected for evidence of joint injury and degeneration at the completion of the study. Articular cartilage surfaces from the medial tibial plateau were examined by light microscopy, the cartilage thickness was measured, and intrinsic material properties were determined by mechanical testing. No joints had ligament or meniscal injuries, cartilage erosions, or osteophytes. Light microscopy did not demonstrate fibrillations in the cartilage. Furthermore, the tibial articular cartilage thickness and mechanical properties did not differ between the exercised group and non-exercised group. These results show that a life time of regular weight bearing exercise in dogs with normal joints did not cause alterations in the structure and mechanical properties of articular cartilage that might lead to joint degeneration.[48] Exercise is healthy and does not cause injury if properly performed. If an injury occurs, it is important to treat it until it is completely healed. The worst things for healing an injury are to take anti-inflammatories or receive cortisone injections. These are the main reasons so many athletes have articular cartilage problems.

Ibuprofen became available over-the-counter in 1955. People have been reaching over the counter ever since then. Sales of over-the-counter pain relievers were $2.67 billion dollars in 1994. There are numerous studies showing the deleterious effects of anti-inflammatories such as Ibuprofen on healing. Ibuprofen, the prototype anti-inflammatory medication, has been shown to have an inhibitory effect on bone healing, remodeling, resorption, and metabolism.[49, 50, 51, 52] Ibuprofen has also been shown to have a tremendous dose-dependent suppressive effect on articular cartilage healing.[53] The higher the Ibuprofen dose, the less healing of the articular cartilage.

Not only is there no evidence that NSAIDs favorably modify the progression of joint breakdown in patients with osteoarthritis or cartilage injury, several NSAIDs, (for example, acetylsalicylic acid (aspirin), Fenoprofen, Tolmetin, and Ibuprofen) have been shown to inhibit the synthesis of proteoglycans by normal cartilage.[54, 55, 56] Because proteoglycans are essential for the elasticity and compressive stiffness of articular cartilage, suppression of their synthesis as a consequence of NSAID administration must have adverse consequences.

NSAIDs inhibit cyclo-oxygenase which is the enzyme involved in the synthesis of prostaglandins which aid in the inflammatory healing response. NSAIDs have the additional effect of inhibiting the enzymes involved in proteoglycan biosynthesis. (**See Figure 8-10.**) Aspirin and Ibuprofen in concentrations that can

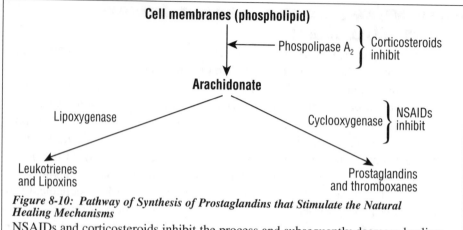

Cell membranes (phospholipid)

Phospolipase A$_2$ } Corticosteroids inhibit

Arachidonate

Lipoxygenase

Cyclooxygenase } NSAIDs inhibit

Leukotrienes and Lipoxins

Prostaglandins and thromboxanes

Figure 8-10: Pathway of Synthesis of Prostaglandins that Stimulate the Natural Healing Mechanisms
NSAIDs and corticosteroids inhibit the process and subsequently decrease healing.

be achieved in joint tissues, inhibit glucuronyltransferase, an enzyme responsible for the elongation of chondroitin sulfate chains on the proteoglycan complex.[57, 58] NSAIDs inhibit the synthesis of proteoglycans that are being made by the chondrocytes to heal the articular cartilage damage.[59] The only result that can be obtained from NSAIDs in a patient with articular cartilage damage is a guarantee to produce more damage. This is exactly what is seen.

When animals with anterior cruciate ligament injuries were given NSAIDs the amount of articular cartilage damage that occurred over time was accelerated at a wicked rate. The proteoglycan concentration of the cartilage matrix was also suppressed significantly.[60, 61]

In 1967, Dr. H. Coke was the first medical doctor to suggest that NSAIDs might accelerate bone destruction.[62] More reports confirmed his suspicions shortly thereafter.[63] In a retrospective study of patients with osteoarthritis of the hip, a variety of NSAIDs were considered to have contributed to destruction of the hip joint confirmed by x-ray studies.[64] Another study confirmed that the stronger the NSAIDs, the faster the arthritic changes occurred.[65] This is why people who start on the anti-inflammatory train need stronger and stronger medications. The NSAIDs accelerate the degenerative process so stronger medications are needed.

For the athlete or the physically active person, the RICE treatment is a scary prospect. It devastates the natural healing response. People are often given NSAIDs along with RICE, which further suppresses the local inflammatory reaction that is needed to heal the injured tissues. Instead of recommending Prolotherapy for continued complaints of pain, the usual course of treatment is perhaps the most potent of all anti-healing therapies: the cortisone shot.

WANT NO BONE? TAKE CORTISONE!

Receiving a cortisone shot is one of the quickest ways to lose strength at the ligament-bone junction (fibro-osseous junction). Cortisone and other steroid shots have the same detrimental effects on articular cartilage healing.

Corticosteroids, such as cortisone and Prednisone, have adverse effects on bone and soft tissue healing. Corticosteroids inactivate vitamin D, limiting calcium absorption by the gastrointestinal tract and increasing the urinary excretion of calcium. Bone also shows a decrease in calcium uptake, ultimately leading to weakness at the fibro-osseous junction. Corticosteroids also inhibit the release of growth hormone, which further decreases soft tissue and bone repair. Ultimately, corticosteroids lead to a decrease in bone, ligament, and tendon strength.[66, 67, 68, 69, 70, 71]

Corticosteroids inhibit the synthesis of proteins, collagen, and proteoglycans, particularly cartilage, by inhibiting chondrocyte production which are the cells that comprise the articular cartilage. The net catabolic effect (weakening) of corticosteroids is inhibition of fibroblast production of collagen, ground substance, and angiogenesis (new blood vessel formation). The result is weakened synovial joints, supporting structures, articular cartilage, ligaments, and tendons. This weakness increases the pain and the increased pain leads to more steroid injections. Cortisone injections should play almost no role in pain management.

Although anti-inflammatory medications and steroid injections reduce pain, they do so at the cost of destroying tissue. In a study conducted by Siraya Chunekamrai, D.V.M., Ph.D., steroid shots were given to horses with a substance commonly used in humans. The injected tissue was examined under the microscope. The steroid shots induced a tremendous amount of damage including chondrocyte necrosis (cartilage cell damage), hypocellularity (decreased number of cells) in the joint, decreased proteoglycan content and synthesis, and decreased collagen synthesis in the joint. All of these effects were permanent.[72]

Dr. Chunekamrai concluded, "The effects on cartilage of intra-articular injections of methylprednisolone acetate (steroid) were not ameliorated at eight weeks after eight weekly injections, or sixteen weeks after a single injection. Cartilage remained biochemically and metabolically impaired."[73] In this study, some of the joints were injected only one time. Even after one steroid injection, cartilage remained biochemically and metabolic impaired. Other studies have confirmed similar harmful effects of steroids on joint and cartilage tissue.[74, 75] A cortisone shot can permanently damage joints. Prolotherapy injections have the opposite effect—they permanently strengthen joints. **Figure 8-11** explains the monumental difference between cortisone and Prolotherapy injections.

Unfortunately, many athletes or people suffering with chronic pain look for quick relief without thinking about the long term, potentially harmful side effects that could occur. The problem with cortisone is that immediate pain relief is possible, but in reality it may be permanently reducing the ability to play sports long-term. Athletes often receive cortisone shots in order to be able to play. They then

PROLOTHERAPY Vs CORTISONE

	PROLOTHERAPY	CORTISONE
EFFECT ON HEALING	Enhanced	Inhibited
EFFECT ON REPAIR	Enhanced	Inhibited
EFFECT ON COLLAGEN GROWTH	Enhanced	Inhibited
EFFECT ON TENDON STRENGTH	Enhanced	Inhibited
EFFECT ON LIGAMENT STRENGTH	Enhanced	Inhibited
EFFECT ON CARTILAGE GROWTH	Enhanced	Inhibited

Figure 8-11: To heal an injury, a person needs to receive Prolotherapy.

go onto the playing field with severe injuries that required cortisone shots to relieve the pain. Because they feel no pain, they play as if the injury does not exist. The injury will unfortunately never heal because of the tremendous anti-healing properties of cortisone. The athlete is therefore further injuring himself by playing. The same goes for the chronic pain sufferer who is trying to be able to return to normal function.

Cortisone is dangerous because it inhibits just about every aspect of healing. Cortisone inhibits prostaglandin and leukotriene productions as already discussed in chapter 7. They also inhibit chondrocyte production of protein polysaccharides (proteoglycans), which are the major constituents of articular ground substance.[76] Behrens and colleagues reported a persistent and highly significant reduction in the synthesis of proteins, collagen, and proteoglycans in the articular cartilage of rabbits who received weekly injections of glucocorticoids. They also reported a progressive loss of endoplasmic reticulum, mitochondria, and Golgi apparatus as the number of injections increased.[77]

THE ROLE OF EXERCISE IN INJURY: RESEARCH WITH EXERCISE AND CORTISONE

Exercise has the opposite effect. Exercise has been shown to positively affect articular cartilage by increasing its thickness, enhancing the infusion of nutrients, and increasing matrix synthesis.[78, 79, 80] However, the effects of both exercise and cortisone in combination were not studied until recently.

In an excellent study pointing out the dangers of an athlete exercising after receiving cortisone, Dr. Prem Gogia and associates at the Washington University School of Medicine in St. Louis, the following was done. Animals were divided into three groups: **1.** Group One received a cortisone shot only. **2.** Group Two received a cortisone shot and exercised, and **3.** Control Group received no treatment. This study was done in 1993 and was the first study to look at the effects of exercising after receiving cortisone shots. The authors did this study because it was common practice in sports medicine to give an athlete with an acute or chronic injury a cortisone shot. Athletes were typically returning to full intensity sports activities within a few hours to one or two days after receiving the shot. The results of the study were amazing.

STUDY RESULTS UNBELIEVABLE

The animals receiving the cortisone shots showed a decrease in chondrocytes. When they exercised in addition to the cortisone shot, the chondrocyte cell count decreased by a full 25 percent. Degenerated cartilage was seen in all the cortisone-injected animals, but severe cartilage damage was seen in 67 percent of the animals that exercised and also received cortisone. The cortisone and exercise group also showed a significant decline in glycosaminoglycan synthesis compared to the other groups. The authors concluded, "The results suggest that running exercise in combination with intra-articular injections results in damage to the femoral articular cartilage." [81]

COMPARISON OF CHANGES IN ARTICULAR CARTILAGE IN AGING AND OSTEOARTHRITIS

CRITERION	AGING	OSTEOARTHRITIS
WATER CONTENT	Decreased	Increased
GLYCOSAMINOGLYCANS		
CHONDROITIN SULFATE	Normal or slightly less	Decreased
GLUCOSAMINE	Increased	Decreased
KERATAN SULFATE	Increased	Decreased
HYALURONATE	Increased	Decreased
PROTEOGLYCANS		
AGGREGATION	Normal	Diminished
LINK PROTEIN	Fragmented	Normal
PROTEASES	"Normal"	Increased

Adapted from **The Biology of Osteoarthritis. Herman, D. The New England Journal of Medicine. 1989, Vol. 20, pp.1322-1329, Table 2**

Figure 8-12 The Joint Composition in Aging and Osteoarthritis are Opposites: Chondroitin and glucosamine content are lower in osteoarthritis. Thus, these patients often require supplementation.

THE CHOICE IS YOURS: OSTEOARTHRITIS OR PROLOTHERAPY?

Osteoarthritis is not the result of aging. **See Figure 8-12**, which dispels the myths about arthritis and aging. The question to then ask is why do most people have arthritis in numerous areas of their body when they are older? Part of the reason for this is that in osteoarthritis, there is a decrease in chondroitin and gluco-somine sulfate levels. This is the basis for their supplementation for this condition.

Otherwise, the answer is simple: Arthritis is the result of an injury to a joint that was never allowed to heal. A normal joint does *not* get arthritis. An aging joint does not get arthritis. An exercised-to-death joint does not get arthritis. *Only an injured joint gets arthritis*. The best way to prevent formation of arthritis—if you participate even in the most brutal of sports such as boxing, martial arts fighting, rugby, or football—is to make sure that your injuries heal. Heal the injury and the likelihood of having a long and prosperous pain-free life is excellent. This means doing the MEAT treatment after the injury. MEAT includes movement, exercise, analgesics, and specific treatments such as heat, ultrasound, massage, and Prolotherapy. Do not allow your injuries to be treated with RICE, anti-inflammatories, cortisone shots, and arthroscopy. If you do these things, the prospects for future arthritis are excellent. The choice is yours: osteoarthritis or Prolotherapy. Perhaps it is for this reason that people around the country are saying no to arthritis and choosing Prolotherapy. ■

Connective Tissue Deficiency: The Underlying Culprit in Chronic Pain and Sports Injury

It is amazing how many chronic pain books rarely mention or do not mention or the words "connective tissue," "ligament," and "collagen." Dysfunctions in these tissues, however, are the cause of almost all chronic pain conditions. By definition when your body feels pain it is telling you that something is wrong. Modern medicine's treatment for acute pain is rest, ice, compression, and elevation (RICE). If this does not work, an anti-inflammatory medication is given. When this does not work, a "stronger, newer, more effective" anti-inflammatory medication is given. When this new medication fails to relieve the pain, cortisone shots are generally given. Traditional orthopedic doctors will then order MRI scans until "the source of the pain" is found. The person is finally subjected to arthroscopes and other surgical procedures to fix the "cartilage" or "disc" problem. The ultimate insult is when the patient is then sent to a "pain specialist" where anti-depressant medications are given because no other cause for the pain but a psychological one can be found. Wouldn't you be depressed if you went through this scenario without resolution of the pain? Sometimes treatments such as biofeedback are tried in order to allow the person to "live with the pain." Eventually diagnoses such as degenerative arthritis or Fibromyalgia are given.

Modern chronic pain management is totally flawed as evidenced by the initial premise that inflammation is the cause of the problem. Inflammation is the natural healing mechanism of the body! Treatments that stimulate inflammation will help relieve the pain and cure people of their painful conditions. Therapies, such as those described above, which stop the normal healing mechanisms of the body, actually promote more injury and pain.

WHAT IS CONNECTIVE TISSUE ANYWAY?

Since healing of chronic pain invariably involves musculoskeletal tissues, a basic knowledge of these tissues is necessary to understand healing. The connective tissues of the body include the muscles, ligaments, tendons, synovium, joint capsules, cartilage, and bones. The connective tissues also involve the ground substance or extracellular matrix around the above mentioned structures. Connective tissue is composed of water, cells such as fibroblasts and chondrocytes, and the substances made by the cells such as collagen and proteoglycans. These substances are what give ligaments, tendons, muscles, joint capsules, discs, and articular cartilage their unique functions and strength.

FIBROBLASTS: THE COLLAGEN BUILDERS

Fibroblasts are crucial for proper healing to occur because they make the collagen, which makes up skin, bone, tendons, ligaments, scars, vessel walls, and viscera and proteoglycans, which make up the connective tissue. Fibroblasts have the capability to replicate in response to injury, growth factors, and inflammatory mediators. Prolotherapy causes fibroblastic proliferation, hence the "prolo" in Prolotherapy, and this is how Prolotherapy stimulates the body (fibroblasts) to repair the painful areas.

CHONDROCYTES: THE CARTILAGE MAKERS

Chondrocytes are responsible for the formation, maintenance, and repair of articular cartilage. From a nutritional viewpoint, chondrocytes are underprivileged cells as they do not have a direct supply of nutrients from blood vessels and depend upon the loading of the joint to push synovial fluid into and out of the interstitial matrix. Like fibroblasts, chondrocytes have the ability to proliferate, but this ability is much more restricted than fibroblasts.

For a long time it was felt that cartilage tissue could not regenerate. Recent research, as well as the successes of Prolotherapy, has proved this notion to be wrong. Chondrocytes, the cells that make collagen and the other components of articular cartilage, gain the ability to replicate, proliferate, and generate new cartilage upon injury.[1,2,3] **(See Figure 9-1.)** This key fact is vital to understanding the power of Prolotherapy in proliferating cartilage. Prolotherapy regenerates cartilage most likely by inducing mature chondrocytes to a chondroblastic state capable of proliferation and repair.

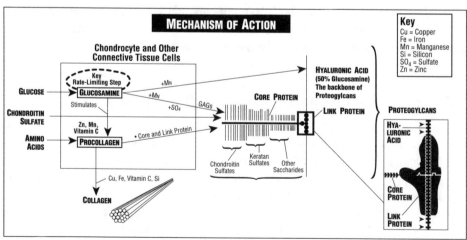

Used with permission from Nutramax Laboratories, Inc.

Figure 9-1: Chondrocytes and Fibroblasts Synthesize Cartilage and Ligaments
Glucosamine and other nutrients are required by the connective tissue cells
to make collagen and proteoglycans, the building blocks of ligaments, tendons
and cartilage.

WATER: CRUCIAL FOR LUBRICATED JOINTS

Connective tissue is comprised of 60 to 80 percent water by weight.[4] Water and proteoglycans provide the lubrication and spacing that are crucial to the gliding function between individual collagen fibers, and give viscoelastic properties to the connective tissue, enabling structures such as ligaments to be strong and somewhat flexible.

A major reason joints stiffen is dehydration. This dehydration factor especially affects the articular cartilage and discs, and is a contributing factor to the great number of people with degenerated discs. Since proteoglycans bind the water in the joints, taking glucosamine and chondroitin sulfate, which are components of proteoglycans, is often recommended for such conditions as arthritis. One of the easiest ways to begin the reversal of connective tissue deficiency is to drink more filtered or distilled water.

PROTEOGLYCANS: THE WATER BINDERS

The proteoglycans are highly viscous proteins that are very hydrophilic, meaning they are attracted to water. The shock-absorbing properties of articular cartilage are primarily due to the proteoglycans. For people with arthritis or athlete's with cartilage damage, a nutritionally-oriented Prolotherapist will recommend oral chondroitin sulfate and glucosamine sulfate. These two substances are components of the articular cartilage that is being repaired. Together with Prolotherapy cartilage will regenerate. Glucosamine can also be added to the Prolotherapy solution and is especially helpful for joints with cartilage deterioration.

COLLAGEN: THE BUILDING BLOCK OF ALL CONNECTIVE TISSUES

Collagen, the major component of connective tissue, comprises seventy to ninety percent of connective tissue weight. Collagen is the most abundant protein in the human body, making up about thirty percent of all proteins.[5] Collagen is the major component of connective tissue, providing tensile strength and structural rigidity to tissues. The synthesis of collagen demands a high amount of amino acids and substrates, as is needed in the formation of any protein. Remember that Prolotherapy just starts the healing process, your body must grow the new tissue. If a person is missing a key amino acid, vitamin, or mineral needed for collagen growth, the proliferation will be incomplete. Caring Medical, our office in Oak Park, IL, has developed some connective tissue products along with the nutritional company, Orthomolecular Products which are given to people undergoing Prolotherapy. This helps ensure that the nutrients and substrates are available to proliferate the collagen and connective tissue repairs.

SOFT TISSUES: MUSCLES, LIGAMENTS AND TENDONS

Whiplash injuries, back strains, ankle sprains, loose joints, and Fibromyalgia, all have as their root cause weakness or deficiency in the soft tissues of the body. These tissues are namely the muscles, tendons, and ligaments. These structures must be repaired and strengthened to cure the chronic pain. One thing most folks know for sure is that the anti-inflammatories, cortisone shots, arthroscopy, and surgery do not repair or strengthen the injured tissues.

The primary function of skeletal muscles is to provide motion and control motion of body parts. One end of the muscle attaches to the bone directly, the other attaches to a tendon, whose main function is to move joints. Ligaments connect bone to bone across joints. Ligaments have more flexibility than tendons and offer passive stabilization of joints when little or no load is applied. The strength of the ligaments around each joint is the determining factor in the joint's overall stability. When the ligaments are injured, they can no longer stabilize the joints, so muscles go into spasm. Chronic muscle spasm is the one of the most sure tail signs of ligament laxity. These chronic muscle spasms cause trigger points in the muscle. These are common in such conditions as myofascial pain syndrome or Fibromyalgia. The most definite treatment to permanently relieve trigger points and chronic muscle tension is Prolotherapy, because only Prolotherapy gets at the root cause of the problem, ligament laxity.

THE CHRONIC PAIN ERROR: LIGAMENTS ARE NOT MUSCLES AND MUSCLES ARE NOT LIGAMENTS

Chronic pain specialists unfortunately fall into the trap that muscles are like ligaments and tendons. As a matter of fact, they are almost exact opposites.

The main difference between muscles and ligaments is that muscles are massively strong structures with a tremendous blood supply. Ligaments, on the other hand, are small tissues that have a poor blood supply. Muscles, because of their good circulation, heal quickly and rarely cause long-term problems. Ligaments on account of their poor blood supply, often heal incompletely and are the cause of most chronic sports injuries and pain. It is our opinion that non-healing ligaments are the number one cause of premature retirement for many athletes and the reason why many people do not enjoy retirement. Ligament laxity is the reason that articular cartilage breaks down and arthritis forms.

Understanding the difference between ligaments and muscles is crucial to understanding why the RICE treatment and anti-inflammatory regimes are totally inappropriate for healing ligaments and why they actually accelerate the degenerative process. **(See Figure 9-2.)** Ligaments, which are generally less than one inch in length, and whose width is measured in millimeters, must be strong because they have the job of binding the bones together. Ligaments owe their great strength to

MUSCLES COMPARED TO LIGAMENTS

	MUSCLES	LIGAMENTS
• FUNCTION	movement	stability
• CIRCULATION BY	large arteries	small arterioles
• BLOOD SUPPLY	excellent	poor
• REPAIR ABILITY	excellent	poor
• CHRONIC INJURIES	rare	high
• APPEARANCE *(BASED ON BLOOD SUPPLY)*	red	white
• SIZE	feet	millimeters
• LOCATION TO JOINTS	outside	inside
• INSERTION SITE	tendons	bone
• COMPARTMENTS	fascial	none
• STRETCHABILITY	good	poor
• INJURY SEVERITY	mild	moderate
• RESPONSE TO EXERCISE	dramatic	little

Figure 9-2: Muscles and ligaments are complete opposites in blood supply, healing ability, and size.

the fact that they are made up of collagen, one of the strongest substances in the human body. Immobility or disuse and the aging process significantly weaken the ligaments. Ligaments normally receive blood vessels from small arterial plexuses from the joints, but they themselves have essentially no blood vessels. This implies that at least some degree of the nutrition must come from diffusion of nutrients, most likely from the joint itself. It should be evident now why ligaments do not repair easily when injured. Because the small blood vessels to the joint are sheared (cut off) during a fall or sports injury; the little blood supply that the ligaments did have is now cut off. The body has to repair the damage, but how can it do so if no immune cells can get to the area because of the poor blood supply? No food, no growth. On top of that, the person puts ice on the area after the injury, which further decreases the blood supply. Eventually anti-inflammatory medications are taken which further decrease the chances the ligament is going to heal. Muscle spasms result because of the instability in the joint due to ligament laxity. *Presto-Change-o*—you now have a chronic pain patient.

An interesting point is that the blood supply to the ligaments is even worse at the point where the ligament attaches to the bone, the fibro-osseous junction. This is the most common area of injury and is responsible for most lingering chronic pains and sports injuries. This is why this exact site is injected with Prolotherapy solution. Okay, the word injection was used! No one likes injections. We don't even like them! We don't even like doctors. But a few minutes of getting injections is a small price to pay to eliminate a lifetime of pain! (**See Figure 9-3.**)

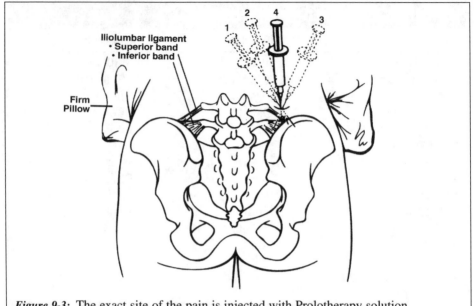

Figure 9-3: The exact site of the pain is injected with Prolotherapy solution.

ARTICULAR CARTILAGE: IT CAN BE REGENERATED

Articular cartilage plays a vital role in the function of the musculoskeletal system by allowing almost frictionless motion to occur between the surfaces of two bones. Furthermore, articular cartilage distributes the load of the joint articulation over a larger contact area, thereby minimizing the contact stresses, and dissipating the energy force associated with the load.

Upon injury, such as mild compression, osteoarthritis, or lacerative injury, these tissues have the ability to heal themselves, yet the notion of damaged cartilage having no regenerative properties is responsible for many people being subjected to arthroscopes with subsequent joint replacements. This falsehood occurs because healthy cartilage cells have very little, if any, mitotic activity—thus very little or no ability to proliferate. That healthy cartilage cells (chondrocytes) have no ability to proliferate and repair was reported in the early 1960's. The first total hip replacement surgery occurred at the same time. A short time later the arthroscope was invented. These occurrences led to the massive proliferation (growth) of the field of orthopedic surgery and numb er of orthopedic surgeons throughout the country. (This is the bad kind of proliferation.)

Since articular cartilage reportedly had no ability to heal, then removal of any damaged articular cartilage was justified. But, as previously noted, articular cartilage does have regenerative properties because the chondrocytes with little regenerative properties themselves revert back to a chondroblastic state, which has tremendous proliferative abilities. This is the probable mechanism by which Prolotherapy acts to induce the regeneration of cartilage. The numerous patients with "no cartilage" who are set for hip/knee replacements but never needed them because of Prolotherapy support this fact.

A good example of this is a patient of ours named Paul. Paul was in his 50's when he came to our Oak Park office with a story heard all too often. He was tremendously athletic in his younger years. He played all of the sports and was even on his college football team. Somewhere in his late teens and early twenties he started getting pain in his lower back and knees. He was given anti-inflammatory medications. This helped for a year or so, at which time he returned to his primary physician to get stronger anti-inflammatory medications. After about eight or ten months, his pain worsened. As he was now out of college holding down a real job, he significantly curbed his sporting events—partly because of time, and partly because of pain. He had some plain x-rays, which showed everything was normal. At this time, he was given his first cortisone shot to relieve the knee pain. This worked for about six months, though his back still gave out occasionally, for which he needed chiropractic care. His orthopedist gave him a referral to physiotherapy of which he completed several courses with only temporary relief of the pain.

"Doctor, it was as if they were not getting at the cause of the pain, only covering it up." Paul sought out the help of massage therapists on his own. "They did more for my pain than any of the doctors." He received several more cortisone shots to his knee when finally the doctor talked him into arthroscopy. This occurred while Paul was in his early 30's. In the meantime his back still hurt.

The arthroscopy of the knee showed some damaged cartilage and meniscus tissue, so it was shaved and removed. This gave him relief for about five years, until the knee pain returned. The pain was then treated with new anti-inflammatory medications. Again, pain relief was provided for about a year, then another new medication was given and so on and so forth. Eventually Paul's whole meniscus was removed. He received a few more cortisone shots and now the doctor was talking about knee replacement! Paul thought, "Forget this noise, there has to be a better answer." He came to our office for a consultation regarding use of Prolotherapy for his condition.

Upon examination, Paul's back was a mess. He had received several rounds of epidural steroid injections with only temporary help. By the time we saw him, his back had already been operated on three times. We looked at his MRI and it was a mess as well. You name the segment of the spine—and there was degeneration. Fortunately for Paul, his proliferative arthritis stopped that day. He was taken off his anti-inflammatory medications and put on a natural medicine program based on his metabolic type. He received Prolotherapy to his knees and lower back.

Over the next few months, Paul received a total of six sessions of Prolotherapy. He now skis, exercises, runs, and lives a vibrant life. Yes, degeneration can stop, but it starts the moment an individual realizes that modern methods of pain control not only do not cure the underlying process, but actually promote it!

CONNECTIVE TISSUE DEFICIENCY SYNDROME

The definition of connective tissue deficiency syndrome is a disorder characterized by a weakening of the connective tissues and a deficiency of the amount or normal functioning of the connective tissues leading to a myriad of painful and chronic symptoms.

Did you ever wonder why your skin gets wrinkles? Why there are bags under your eyes? Why your skin is sagging under the chin and arms? Why your joints get puffy, aching, and cracking? Why your nails and hair are dull and brittle? Why you get skin growths? Why you get more exhausted and sore from exercise as you get older? Why doctors cannot figure out why you are so tired, have allergies, and cannot get rid of your chronic pain?

The answer is easy. Doctors simply do not receive training in nutritional, connective tissue, and ligament problems, and thus never properly diagnose connective tissue deficiencies. How can you know that you have a connective tissue problem? Do you have any of the conditions noted below? Has anyone ever given you any of the following diagnoses?

- Allergies
- Coronary artery disease
- Myofascial pain syndrome
- Leaky-gut syndrome
- Chronic fatigue syndrome
- Non-healing sports injury
- Premature gray
- Endocrine insufficiencies
- Fibromyalgia
- Ulcerative colitis
- Periodontal disease
- Asthma
- Arthritis
- Chronic pain syndrome
- Eczema
- Acne
- Immunodeficiency
- Interstitial cystitis
- Premature aging
- Loose joints
- Crohns disease
- Immune dysfunction
- Macular degeneration
- Other chronic degenerative diseases

All of these conditions have an association with connective tissue deficiency as their root cause.

DIAGNOSING CONNECTIVE TISSUE DEFICIENCY

The breakdown of collagen leads to the systemic release of hydroxyproline, an amino acid primarily exclusive to collagen. Research done at our office, Caring Medical and Rehabilitation Services in Oak Park, and other studies have shown that by measuring free and peptide-bound hydroxyproline, as well as hydroxyproline levels in the urine after a course of strenuous exercise, these markers for connective tissue deficiency syndrome can be seen. On physical examination things such as excessive looseness of the skin, frail dull hair, and the individual medical history give signs that the person has lost the ability to repair or regenerate connective tissue.

SOLVING CONNECTIVE TISSUE DEFICIENCY

Prevention is always the best medicine. If a person is injured, the MEAT protocol is performed to stimulate soft tissue healing. This involves movement, exercise, analgesics, and specific treatments such as ultrasound, heat, massage, physiotherapy and possibly Prolotherapy. Unfortunately, most people who sprain ankles and professional athletes who are injured in a game do the exact opposite of MEAT and halt the body's chance to heal the soft tissue injuries because they use RICE treatments instead of MEAT treatment. RICE stands for rest, ice, compression, and elevation. RICE means immobility and ice, both of which mean bad news for connective tissues. The RICE protocol, including cortisone and anti-inflammatory medications, has the following effects on connective tissue healing:

RICE VERSUS MEAT:	RICE	MEAT
● Capillary vasoconstriction (cut off blood supply):	Increased	Decreased
● Blood flow	Decreased	Increased
● Migration of immune cells to the area	Decreased	Increased
● New blood vessel formation	Decreased	Increased
● Fibroblast proliferation (growth)	Decreased	Increased
● Deposition of collagen	Decreased	Increased
● Collagen strength	Decreased	Increased
● Protein synthesis of regenerating tissue	Decreased	Increased
● Ligament and tendon strength	Decreased	Increased
● Cartilage breakdown	Increased	Decreased
● Proteoglycan synthesis	Decreased	Increased
● Collagen synthesis by fibroblasts	Decreased	Increased

Figure 9-4: Comparison of RICE Vs. MEAT Treatment in Healing Connective Tissue Deficiency. Which makes the most sense to you?

To have any chance to heal soft tissue injuries and be cured of chronic pain, the use of anti-inflammatory medications and cortisone shots must be stopped and Prolotherapy begun. Prolotherapy can be done while a patient is taking anti-inflammatories, but it will take longer to heal. Pain relief with Prolotherapy generally comes immediately, with 67 percent of people feeling better after the very first treatment. Switching from anti-inflammatory medications to Ultram (a non-narcotic pain reliever with no anti-inflammatory activity) is also a good idea if pain medication is needed. The patient will likely not need the Ultram for very long. Tylenol may also be used because its anti-inflammatory effects are generally negligible.

If a person suffering from chronic pain exhibits evidence of systemic inflammation, such as being tender all over, most likely a diagnosis of Fibromyalgia or a rheumatological disease has already been given. In such a case high dose proteolytic enzymes like bromelain and omega-3 fatty acids such as EPA/DHA in the form of cod liver oil are generally given. Other oils such as evening primrose oil, borage oil, and flax seed oil may also be used. These are typically necessary when weaning someone off of anti-inflammatory medications. At Caring Medical and Rehabilitation Services we set up individual protocols to help wean the patient from high dose Prednisone and other steroids. Even people with rheumatoid arthritis can be cured of rheumatoid arthritis with natural remedies. Yes, not only is it possible to get rid of Prednisone and relieve pain by treating the connective tissue deficiency, but these people can actually test rheumatoid factor negative in the blood, thus proving the condition is indeed cured.

CATABOLIC VERSUS ANABOLIC: WHICH ARE YOU?

If you are a person with chronic pain and reading this book about this crazy-sounding injection treatment, you are most likely catabolic. Catabolic refers to the fact that your body is in a state of breakdown (a nicer way than saying you are decaying). Of course, you would prefer to be anabolic, or having your body be in a state of being built up, regenerated, or repaired. A person with connective tissue deficiency is in a catabolic state and the only way to cure the chronic pain is to become anabolic.

The following hormones are very anabolic in regards to helping stimulate connective tissue: Growth Hormone, DHEA, testosterone, and progesterone. What most people do not realize is that estrogen, especially estradiol, has very catabolic effects on connective tissue. Perhaps this is one time where the phrase "be a man" may be a good thing. Ladies, that's a joke!

It was always interesting why most chronic pain clinics are filled with women. Even women athletes are much more likely to become injured than their male counterparts in the same sports.[6] The answer to both of these mysteries is explained by the fact that the female hormone estradiol inhibits collagen synthesis by inhibiting fibroblastic proliferation. Estrogen is known to increase the deposition of fat in the female, especially in certain tissues such as the breast, hips, and subcutaneous tissues. This perhaps also explains the fact that most men "age gracefully" and often women do not.

In a landmark study, published in 1998, researchers at the UCLA School of Medicine studied the effect of estradiol on the cellular proliferation and collagen synthesis of fibroblasts derived from the anterior cruciate ligament.[7] Their findings are seen in **Figures 9-5 and 9-6.**

A significant reduction of fibroblast proliferation was observed with increasing estradiol concentrations. Within normal physiologic levels of estrogen, collagen synthesis was reduced by more than 40 percent of controls, and at pharmacological levels of estrogen (women taking birth control pills and post-menopausal synthetic hormone replacement); collagen proliferation was inhibited by 50 percent. **It is probable that women are much more likely than men to suffer from**

the effects of connective tissue deficiency, especially as it pertains to having chronic pain because of higher estrogen levels. Many other researchers have found similar inhibitory effects of estradiol on connective tissue proliferation.[8, 9, 10]

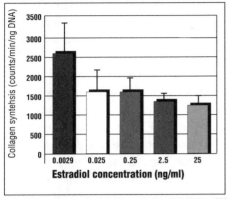

Adapted from *American Journal of Sports Medicine Vol. 25, Page 707*
©1998

Figure 9-5: Collagen Synthesis is inhibited by Increased Estradiol Levels.

Progesterone, the other female hormone, in many respects has the opposite effects of estrogen. Progesterone has been shown to stimulate collagen proliferation and decrease collagen breakdown.[11, 12] It is also known as a bone-trophic hormone by its ability to stimulate osteoblastic activity and thus stimulate bone growth and combat osteoporosis.[13, 14, 15]

Many, many women are estrogen dominant, meaning they have too much estradiol and not enough progesterone. The cure for this, like modern medicine's cure for everything, is pills. This time we are talking about birth control pills. Oral contraceptive pills (the politically correct name) are just a cover-up for the biochemical abnormality causing the estrogen dominance in the woman. Why do you think breast cancer is so much on the rise? Why do so many women have PMS with its irritability, bloating, and severe menstrual cramps? Estrogen excess can also cause migraine headaches, Fibromyalgia, and of course, general chronic pain.

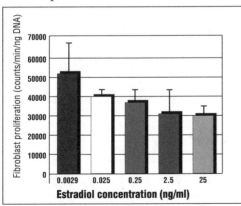

Adapted from *American Journal of Sports Medicine Vol. 25, Page 707*
©1998

Figure 9-6: Fibroblast proliferation is inhibited by Increased Estradiol Levels.

A better course of action for women with connective tissue deficiency due to estrogen excess is first to document it. A full comprehensive hormone panel including estradiol, progesterone, DHEA, testosterone, IGF-1 (marker for Growth Hormone) and thyroid is ideal. The next step is to undergo a nutritional evaluation to determine which foods are best to eat. Caring Medical in Oak Park, Illinois, does Metabolic Typing which takes into account the following factors: oxidative rate of food, blood/urine/saliva pH, body

type and few other variables in determining the proper diet. This then helps change a women's physiology so she does not produce so much estrogen and her estradiol to progesterone levels become more balanced.

115

A good sign that a woman's hormones are balanced is a regular menstrual cycle with no cramping or PMS, and a normal menstruation. For the woman who has cramping, bloating, PMS, excessive flow, and an irregular cycle, excessive estrogen is most likely. Often diagnostic testing in such an individual finds that the diet is full of simple carbohydrates, including excessive sugars, fruit juice, and white flour or wheat. Cutting back on the breads, pastas, and sugar is a good idea. The other metabolic abnormality that is found is an essential fatty acid deficiency. This is corrected by increasing the amounts of omega-3 fatty acids in the diet as is found in fresh fish (especially fish with scales). Supplementing with the omega-3 fatty acids, eicosapentaenoic and docosahexaenoic acid, which are found in cod liver oil, are also beneficial. Other recommendations to help balance a woman's hormones to be more pro-connective tissue growth are to increase the protein in the diet especially with soy products. Soy is one of the specific nutrients and herbal supplements that can reduce estrogen bioavailability in females.[16] Other phytoestrogens (plant based products with some estrogenic qualities) include alfalfa and the Chinese herb angelica sinesis or Dong Quai. Two herbs that have specifically been shown to directly reduce estradiol levels are *urtica dioica* (stinging nettles) and *vitex agnus castus* (chaste berry). [17 18] Specific herbal products that we use at Caring Medical and Rehabilitation Services to combat connective tissue deficiency are described later.

The woman with chronic pain and connective tissue deficiency that is not being completely resolved with the dietary and herbal recommendations above, may need to take some natural progesterone, or other anabolic hormones that stimulate connective tissue proliferation. Of course, the most powerful of all the connective tissue proliferants is Prolotherapy directly into the site of pain. The more anabolic your hormonal milieu, the better the response to Prolotherapy and the more likely that pain will be cured permanently. If Prolotherapy relieves the pain, only to have it recur a year or so later, this is a sign that the body is in a catabolic state. To permanently cure the pain, not only will Prolotherapy be given, but it will also be necessary to assess and then correct the hormonal imbalances.

ANABOLISM: THE ONLY CHANCE TO CURE CHRONIC PAIN

When asked the question, "Do you want a treatment that weakens your body or strengthens it?" You can bet that most people would choose a treatment that strengthens the body. The next question to ask is, "Why do you take anti-inflammatories and cortisone shots?" It makes you shudder when a person comes to the office with a history of having four different joints surgerized, arthritis throughout the body, and wanting us to cure their knee pain without monkeying with their pain pills! This is a ludicrous request because the anti-inflammatory pain pills most likely got them into this state in the first place! Anti-inflammatory medications stop the natural healing processes of the body, so the body becomes more catabolic or stops healing and starts breaking down. The only chance such an individual has to cure the chronic pain is for the body to become anabolic. Do this and receive Prolotherapy and the prognosis goes from critical to optimistic! The primary compounds responsible for building up the connective tissues in the body are the anabolic hormones including DHEA, testosterone, and Growth Hormone and its associated growth factor, IGF-1.

DHEA: THE ADRENAL GLAND'S MASTER HORMONE

Dehydroepiandrosterone is a steroid hormone secreted by the adrenal gland in quantities twenty-fold greater than any other adrenal steroid. DHEA levels, like other anabolic hormone levels, decline rapidly with age in both men and women after the age of thirty—yikes that includes us! **(See Figures 9-7 and 9-8.)**

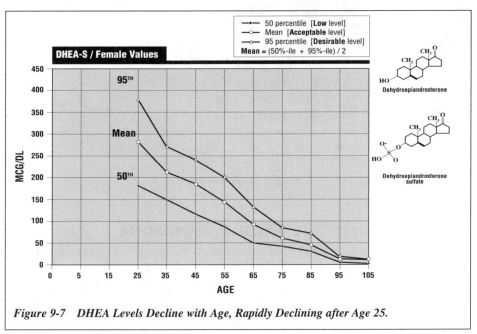

Figure 9-7   DHEA Levels Decline with Age, Rapidly Declining after Age 25.

Adapted from AMTL Corporation's Natural Progesterone: The Multiple Roles of a Remarkable Hormone *by John R. Lee*

Current research suggests that DHEA may be of value in preventing and treating cardiovascular disease, high cholesterol, diabetes, obesity, cancer, memory disturbances, immune system disorders and chronic fatigue. DHEA is probably so potent because it causes a significant rise in IGF-1 levels, a marker for Growth Hormone.[19] DHEA itself has trophic effects including bone and connective tissue building.[20] As a matter of fact, one of the most amazing findings with DHEA is that chronic joint pains and immobility improve with its supplementation. DHEA also helps connective tissue deficiency by stimulating immune function. DHEA reverses the negative effects that cortisone and other glucocorticosteroids have on suppressing the immune system. DHEA is impor-

because the beneficial effects of Prolotherapy are dependent on a well-functioning immune system. The stronger the immune system, the stronger the response to Prolotherapy.

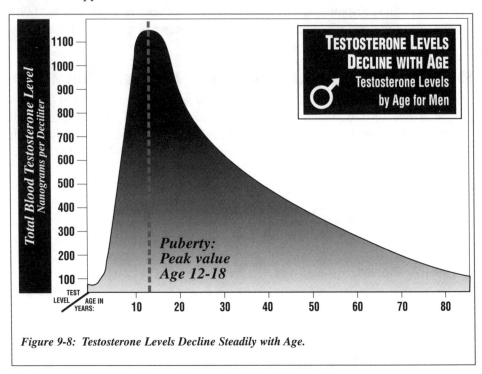

Figure 9-8: Testosterone Levels Decline Steadily with Age.

TESTOSTERONE: THE MANLY HORMONE

It is always funny to see the reaction of most women when testosterone is recommended. They often say, "I don't want to get a beard, are you nuts?!" You bet we're nuts. We're nuts about getting you better. Men secrete many times more testosterone than women, so the dose for replacing a woman's testosterone is much less. Yes, you heard us right, replacing a woman's testosterone. Women make testosterone and need it to build connective tissue so they look younger, have less fat, keep skin healthy, repair connective tissues better, and improve the sex drive. Besides its obvious effects, testosterone has anabolic or tissue-building properties that are beneficial in wound healing and stimulating bone and connective tissue growth. You know this is true because men have 40 to 50 percent more muscle than women.

Testosterone has been shown to totally reverse the negative effects of estradiol on the proliferation of type III collagen.[21] It is important to realize that the primary event in the start of post-menopausal osteoporosis is the loss of collagen. This is why Growth Hormone (IGF-1) and testosterone are so important because they provide the most stimulatory effects on collagen and bone production. This is why osteoporosis is very rare in males. The testosterone they continue to produce preserves their bone structure as well as their connective tissue. Men who lack testosterone develop osteoporosis and chronic pain.

Women secrete testosterone and other male hormones, as they are vital to a woman's health. Testosterone does many other things that benefit women and helps us convince them to take it. Testosterone stimulates collagen growth throughout the body including the hair, nails, and skin. Who doesn't want thicker hair, skin, and nails? Testosterone also increases the basal metabolic rate by as much as 15 percent.[22] This helps people who take it loose weight, but gain muscle mass. Problems occur when these anabolic hormone levels become too low and cause connective tissue deficiency. This typically occurs after menopause for women, when androgen production decreases by as much as 50 percent. It is for this reason that women with connective tissue problems need to think about taking natural testosterone, androgenic herbs, or stimulating testosterone production through diet. Testosterone helps the body retain muscle and protein, and thus it is stimulated by a high protein diet.[23] Two herbal remedies that have been shown to increase testosterone availability are Panax ginseng and *cinnamomum cassia.* Thus, increasing the protein in the diet (yes, more eggs, chicken, fish, nuts, seeds, and tofu), taking Panax ginseng, along with natural testosterone are often part of the program to reverse connective tissue deficiency and eliminate chronic pain.

GROWTH HORMONE: IT LIVES UP TO ITS NAME!

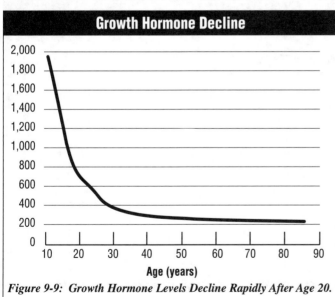

Figure 9-9: Growth Hormone Levels Decline Rapidly After Age 20.

The most abundant hormone made by the master endocrine gland, the pituitary gland, is Growth Hormone. Growth Hormone, once it hits the blood stream, only lasts a few minutes. This is enough time to stimulate its uptake into the liver, where it is converted into growth factors. The most important of these is Insulin-like Growth Factor 1 (IGF-1), also known as somatomedin C.

Growth Hormone declines with age, the level of Growth Hormone after the ages of 21 to 31 falling about 14 percent per decade. By age 60 the Growth Hormone production rate is reduced by half. This is extremely significant because besides its general effect in causing growth, Growth Hormone has many specific metabolic effects as well, including **1.** increased rate of protein synthesis in all cells of the body; **2.** increased mobilization of fatty acids from adipose tissue, increased free fatty acids in the blood, and increased use of the fatty acids for energy; and **3.** decreased rate of glucose utilization throughout the body.[24] Thus, in effect, Growth Hormone enhances the body protein, uses up the fat stores, and conserves carbohydrate. **Figure 9-10** shows some of the beneficial effects for people taking Growth Hormone.

The more you learn about Growth Hormone and its growth factor IGF-1, the more you want it! Growth hormone is used medically to stimulate collagen growth especially for poor healing wounds like burns. Injections of Growth Hormone

EFFECTS OF GROWTH HORMONE ADMINISTRATION

STRENGTH, EXERCISE & BODY FAT	IMPROVEMENT
Muscle strength	88%
Muscle size	81%
Body fat loss	72%
Exercise tolerance	81%
Exercise endurance	83%

SKIN & HAIR	
Skin texture	71%
Skin thickness	68%
Skin elasticity	71%
Wrinkle disappearance	51%
New hair growth	38%

HEALING, FLEXIBILITY & RESISTANCE	
Healing of old injuries	55%
Healing of other injuries	61%
Healing capacity	71%
Back flexibility	53%
Resistance to common illness	73%

SEXUAL FUNCTION	
Sexual potency/frequency	75%
Duration of penile erection	62%
Frequency of night time urination	57%
Hot flashes	58%
Menstrual cycle regulation	39%

ENERGY, EMOTIONS & MEMORY	
Energy level	84%
Emotional stability	67%
Attitude toward life	78%
Memory	62%

Adapted from Growth Hormone, Reversing Human Aging Naturally by James Jamieson

Figure 9-10: The Beneficial Effects of Growth Hormone Administration
Improvement in strength, exercise tolerance, body fat, skin, hair, healing, sexual function, and energy in a study involving 202 patients is shown with Growth Hormone.

stimulate the formation of collagen, increase the tensile strength of wounds, and make wounds heal faster. Growth Hormone directly stimulates protein synthesis everywhere in the body, but especially in the connective tissues.[25, 26]

Growth Hormone's effects on connective tissues are probably mediated through IGF-1 since specific receptors for this growth factor are present on fibroblasts and osteoblasts.[27, 28] IGF-1 has been shown to directly stimulate collagen synthesis and replication of these cells.[29, 30] As it turns out estradiol is apparently a potent inhibitor of IGF-1 secretion, and this fact is probably the mechanism upon which estradiol inhibits connective tissue proliferation.[31]

"Doctor, I beg you, please show me why my Growth Hormone levels are low." This question is vital to curing chronic pain and enhancing athletic performance because Growth Hormone is the primary stimulator of connective tissue proliferation. Growth Hormone, as it turns out, is secreted in a pulsatile manner and increases and decreases within minutes. The surges of secretion occur at three- to five-hour intervals with the greatest surge in young individuals occurring 60 to 90 minutes after the onset of deep sleep. Insomnia or sleep deprivation is one of the most potent inhibitors of Growth Hormone secretion.[32] **(See Figure 9-11.)**

Besides deep sleep the other stimulators of Growth Hormone secretion include: starvation, hypoglycemia, low free fatty acids in the blood, exercise, excitement, and trauma.[33] Because starvation is a potent stimulator of Growth Hormone, one of the best things a person with chronic pain can do is not eat after dinner. Yes, no more late night rendezvous with the refrigerator! The person who undergoes a vigorous work-out, goes to bed on an empty stomach, and gets a real deep sleep for six hours is giving the body an optimal state for con-

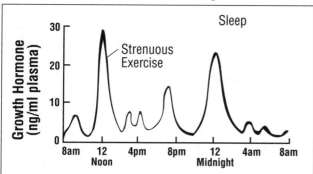

Figure 9-11: Growth Hormone Secretion Occurs in Peaks
Adapted from *Textbook of Medical Physiology*, by A. Guyton and J. Hall, © 1996, W.B. Saunders Co., Philadelphia

nective tissue proliferation through enhancing Growth Hormone secretion. This explains what happens in such conditions as Fibromyalgia. The person suffers an injury and it causes pain. The pain then causes non-restful sleep. The non-restful sleep inhibits Growth Hormone secretion, so the body goes into a catabolic state because of low Growth Hormone levels. The body cannot repair the connective tissues, therefore they become weaker and injured. There you have it, diffuse body pain. Sound familiar? If this sounds like we are describing you, run to your nearest Prolotherapist who does natural medicine and start stimulating the growth of your connective tissues.

The wonderful thing about Growth Hormone is that it is secreted primarily during stage three and stage four sleep, which are deep sleep cycles. To encourage Growth Hormone production, all you have to do is get deeper nights' sleep. To help this production, deep sleep-inducing agents are often given. Natural herbal remedies such as passion flower, valerian root, blue vervain, hops, and chamomile are tried first. For the person with chronic pain and insomnia these are usually not strong enough so that more potent natural sleep-inducing agents such as tryptophan and gamma hydroxybutyrate are given. The one that we have had the best success with is gamma hydroxybutyrate (GHB). GHB is a neurotransmitter that is involved in the regulation of the anterior pituitary gland, which secretes Growth Hormone. In some studies Growth Hormone secretion has increased sixteen fold with the use of this substance.[34] Caring Medical also uses products that stimulate GHB production in the body. It is imperative for the person with chronic pain to get at least six hours of deep sleep to be in optimal shape to restore health!

Because Growth Hormone is secreted at night, natural remedies to induce its secretion are taken at night. There are many different secretagogues that natural medicine physicians use to induce Growth Hormone secretion. There are also various amino acids including arginine, lysine, glutamine, ornithine, alpha-ketoglutarate, and glycine, which have various properties that raise Growth Hormone production. The specific products used at Caring Medical in Oak Park, Illinois will be discussed in the next few pages.

In an ideal setting, the person with chronic pain and connective tissue deficiency would monitor the Growth Hormone (IGF-1) levels as supplementation is given. Low levels are supplemented with natural medicine protocols to improve the levels. By inducing deep sleep and taking supplements to raise IGF-1 levels, you will be well on your way to relieving your chronic pain and sports injuries, because your body will have perhaps the most systemic promoter of connective tissue growth: Growth Hormone. For those who can afford it, injections of the actual Growth Hormone can be done at home. This is the most direct way to raise your Growth Hormone levels. It is also the easiest way to "grow young." Growth Hormone does what its name implies: grows tissue. Connective tissue proliferation is what you need to permanently eliminate chronic pain!

PROLOTHERAPY: PROLIFERATING THE EXACT SITE OF THE PAIN

Prolotherapy is the only treatment that stimulates the body to repair the painful area exactly at the site of the injury. Prolotherapy injections of natural substances stimulate fibroblastic growth to proliferate collagen tissue exactly at the site of pain where the ligaments and tendons attach to the bone called the fibro-osseous junction. **(See Figure 9-12.)** Immediately after the injections, there will be slight pain and swelling at the site, confirming that the natural healing inflammatory process has begun. There are generally about one to two days of soreness after

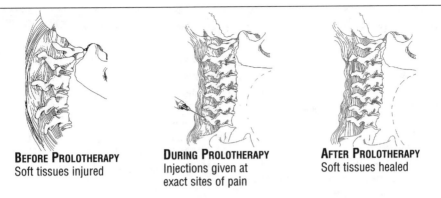

BEFORE PROLOTHERAPY	DURING PROLOTHERAPY	AFTER PROLOTHERAPY
Soft tissues injured	Injections given at exact sites of pain	Soft tissues healed

Figure 9-12: Prolotherapy Curing Neck Pain from Any Musculoskeletal Cause
Prolotherapy stimulates the growth of soft tissue, such as ligaments and tendons, relieving chronic neck pain.

Prolotherapy. If the soreness lasts longer than this, it is not a bad sign—it just means that more inflammation has been produced, which means that more connective tissue will be produced. Prolonged stiffness can therefore be a very good sign. If the stiffness causes too much pain, a mild analgesic and massage therapy to the area is recommended.

If your body is in an anabolic state, then the likelihood of completely relieving your chronic pain is excellent. In such an instance, generally just four to six treatments are needed per area. The treatments are generally given every four to six weeks to allow sufficient time for the connective tissue to grow.

Prolotherapy in conjunction with treating systemic connective deficiency syndromes, as described above, can have dramatic results even in severe cases. Many people have come to our office saying that they were told their cases were hopeless. Fortunately there is a cure for chronic pain and sports injuries, and that cure is Prolotherapy.

CONNECTIVE TISSUE DEFICIENCY HAS MANY CAUSES

There are hundreds of factors that affect connective tissue healing including age, types of tissue injured, circulation, medications, and many others as depicted in **Figure 9-13**. The most important of these are the nutritional status and medical condition of the person. People who consume very healthy diets, eat according to their Metabolic Types, and have no systemic medical conditions, have an excellent chance to heal their chronic pains with Prolotherapy. If they experience positive jump signs where tendons or ligaments attach to the bones, then they have almost a one hundred percent chance of curing their chronic pain with Prolotherapy. Other doctors might give a more conservative answer at eighty-five percent. For the people who consume unhealthy diets and who have systemic medical conditions that harm soft tissue healing, the chance of healing with Prolotherapy declines. This should not discourage these people because just

FACTORS AFFECTING HEALING OF CONNECTIVE TISSUES

- Age
- Gender
- Type of Injury
- Severity of injury
- Underlying disease processes
- Hormonal influences
- Dietary intake
- Nutritional status
- Degree of hypoxia (systemic and local)
- Type of tissue(s) affected
- Electrical fields
- Mechanical load forces
- Temperature
- Pharmacological agents (drugs)

- Mobility (local & whole body)
- Type of onset (acute or chronic)
- Structural (physical) deformities
- Psychological influences (placebo effects and psychoneuroimmunological links)
- Metabolic and cell turnover rates of connective tissues
- Muscular strength and forces
- Blood supply
- Overall health status
- Timing and return to physical activity
- pH and lactate concentration
- Growth factors, cytokines, eicosanoids

Adapted from *Nutrition Applied to Injury Rehabilitation and Sports Medicine* by Bucci, L. CRC Press, Boca Raton FL © 1995

Figure 9-13: Factors Affecting the Healing of Connective Tissue

about every medical condition can be improved with natural medicine remedies and techniques to move a person from the good to excellent Prolotherapy candidate category.

To enhance the healing from Prolotherapy, several nutritional products were designed to enhance connective tissue proliferation by the combined efforts of Caring Medical in Oak Park, Illinois and Ortho Molecular Products in Plover, Wisconsin. These products are vitamins/minerals/herbal combinations designed to help stimulate connective tissue proliferation and reverse the effects of connective tissue deficiency. They are as follows:

- **Ortho Prolo Max:** This product includes ginseng, RNA, L-proline, glucosamine, and horsetail. It is used as a first-line supplement for such conditions as acute injury, Fibromyalgia, and as a post-Prolotherapy supplement to aid healing.

- **Ortho Derma:** This product includes vitamins A, D, E, as well as zinc, silica, gotu kola, and nettles leaf. It is used for connective tissue deficiency where obvious skin abnormalities are seen including excessive wrinkles, bags under the eyes, dryness, or acne.

- **Cosmedix:** This product includes biotin, selenium, betaine, para-aminobenzoic acid, as well as MSM. It is used for connective tissue deficiency where signs are prevalent in the hair and nails. This could be in the form of brittle nails/hair, excessive lines in the nails, split ends, dull hair, or loosing hair.

● **Vessel Max:** this product contains horsechestnut, butchers broom, gotu kola, and troxerutin. It is used for vascular connective tissue deficiency as evidenced by spider or varicose veins, or where there is a history of an aneurysm.

People desiring to reverse connective tissue deficiency through nutrition and nutritional supplements may benefit from some or all of the above products. Patients with connective tissue deficiency in addition to excessive weight problems, use the Ortho Lean program, which includes Lean Product Meal Replacement, Daytime Lean Enhancer, Nighttime Lean Enhancer, and of course, The Dr. and Dietitian booklet. These products are not just designed to help you lose weight, but to lose fat, gain muscle and other beneficial connective tissue. They do this by providing the precursors to form and stimulate connective tissue growth by enhancing Growth Hormone secretion. Perhaps the most exciting products that have been developed are those in the sports product line. Athletes, by the very nature of their activities, are continually breaking down connective tissues. Most athletes are not on any nutritional program, let alone one that is complete. Thus we saw the need to develop the Ortho Sports Line. Besides having products that enhance muscle formation, there are those that speed up recovery time, reduce post-exercise muscle soreness, and enhance speed. They do this all by reversing connective tissue deficiency. To cure chronic pain and help ensure no relapses, the health of the connective tissues must take first priority.

To learn more about the nutrients needed to proliferate connective tissues please read the next book to be released by Beulah Land Press: *The Chronic Disease Cure! Reversing Chronic Degenerative Diseases through Connective Tissue Proliferation,* by Ross and Marion Hauser. (Due out late 2000.)

To obtain information on the above products designed specifically to reverse connective tissue deficiency, as well as the other products designed by OrthoMolecular Products:

ORTHOMOLECULAR PRODUCTS
2771 CEDAR DRIVE
P.O. BOX 520
PLOVER, WI 54467
1-800-332-2351

To order the products directly, call

BEULAH LAND NUTRITIONALS
708-848-7789

and ask to speak to someone in the pharmacy.

■

Nutrition and Chronic Pain

Congratulations! You have made it this far in the book. We hope you enjoyed it. Now you know why ligament and tendon weakness is commonly the cause of chronic pain and what can be done about it.

Prolotherapy starts the growth of ligament and tendon tissue, but you grow the tissue. If you stock your body with all the nutrients available—amino acids, vitamins, minerals, and essential fatty acids—optimum health and strong tissue will be the result.

Many people do not realize that a lunch salad does not provide them with three weeks worth of nutrition. A patient once replied when asked how many vegetable servings he consumed per day, "Three."

"Really? What do you eat?"

"Well, for lunch I usually have a hamburger. There is ketchup, tomato, and onion on it. That's three vegetables."

Unfortunately, condiments and hamburger toppings are not complete vegetable servings.

THE IMPORTANCE OF NUTRITION

Nutrients, like minerals and most vitamins, are water soluble. Consequently, whatever the body does not need for that day will be excreted in the urine. Therefore, vitamins and minerals need to be consumed daily to achieve optimum health. In their food pyramid, the United States government recommends consuming two to four servings of fruit and three to five servings of vegetables per day. The dietary habits of most Americans fall far short of meeting these recommendations.

During the past 40 years, the amount of nutrition in food products has declined largely due to poor soil quality. Today, it is very difficult to obtain adequate daily nutrients even when strictly adhering to the food pyramid. Manure is no longer used as fertilizer and the land is never given a chance to rest. An apple today does not have the same nutrient value apples did 40 years ago. Organic apples fertilized with manure are more nutritious than apples grown with chemical fertilizers and sprayed with pesticides. We strongly recommend organic foods. Besides their nutritional value, organically grown foods do not contain the chemical toxins found in conventionally grown foods.

Vitamin and mineral supplements, especially a general multivitamin, will aid you in your quest to obtain enough daily nutrients. Other specific nutrients may be helpful, depending on your health. If you seek preventative care from a Natural Medicine physician and develop an interest in nutrition, you will soon be on the road to wellness.

A SUPPLEMENT TO PROMOTE HEALING

People receiving Prolotherapy treatments often ask if there are supplements they should take to aid in the healing of their ligaments and tendons. The first step would be to undergo Metabolic Typing to individually determine what foods will contribute to the healing process. The next step would be to take a good general vitamin and mineral supplement.

A supplement that we formulated for Orthomolecular Products that is specifically designed to help grow ligament and tendon tissue is called Ortho Prolo Max, has unique ingredients that have been shown to help collagen formation in the body. Ortho Prolo Max contains the following ingredients:

INGREDIENTS:	REASON:
L-PROLINE	COLLAGEN IS ONE-THIRD PROLINE
L-CYSTEINE	CRITICAL TO SOFT TISSUE HEALING
GRAPE SEED PROCYANADINS	NATURAL ANTIOXIDANT
GLUCOSAMINE SULFATE	A COMPONENT OF TENDON AND LIGAMENT TISSUE
HORSETAIL HERB	NATURAL SOURCE OF SILICA
RNA	HELP FIBROBLASTS (WHICH GROW COLLAGEN) REPLICATE
CENTELLA ASIATICA HERB	ENHANCES CONNECTIVE TISSUE STRUCTURE
MSM (METHYLSULFONYLMETHANE)	NATURAL SOURCE OF SULFUR

The product also contains other ingredients that we feel help soft tissue heal, thereby aiding Prolotherapy treatments. We have also formulated other products designed to enhance connective tissue proliferation. These include Ortho Derma, Cosmedix, Vessel Max—all produced by Orthomolecular Products.

Lastly, specific nutrients may be added depending on an individual's needs. If someone appears to be tired, Ginseng, Licorice Root, or other nutrients for adrenal support may be added. If muscle spasms are a major issue then more magnesium, calcium, or potassium may be added. The Metabolic Typing will also give some indication that other nutrients are needed. Don't wait until you are sick. Prevent sickness by paying attention to your health now.

METABOLIC TYPING

At our Natural Medicine clinic in Oak Park, Illinois, we use a laboratory test called Metabolic Typing to determine specific nutritional needs. Metabolic Typing is a process that determines a person's basic underlying physiology. In simplistic terms, some people have the physiology of a lion and others have that of a giraffe. No, it does not mean some people are hairy and others have long necks. A lion survives best on a high protein diet, whereas a giraffe fares better on a vegetarian-based diet. Metabolic Typing can determine which type of nutritional program best suits a particular individual and what vitamins and minerals are needed.

127

Metabolic Typing involves monitoring a patient's detailed diet history with subsequent general well-being after they eat various foods. Lion metabolic types tend to feel better after eating meat, chicken, fish, and other foods high in protein. Giraffe metabolic types feel better after consuming salad, fruit, vegetables, pasta, coffee, and tea.

Lions generally have acid blood, alkaline urine, and are called acid blood types. Giraffes generally have alkaline blood, acid urine, and are called alkaline blood types. The acid-alkaline terminology refers to the pH of the various body fluids. Acid pH means the pH is lower than normal, whereas alkaline pH means the pH is higher than normal.

In order to determine a metabolic type, the patient provides urine, saliva, and blood samples after having fasted for 15 hours and at one-and-a-half hours after eating a meal. The pH of each fluid is tested. Other tests are done on the urine sample to provide a "metabolic picture" of the patient's body functions, as described by Carey Reams, Ph.D.[1] The patient is then given a 50-gram glucose fruit drink and fingerstick blood sugars are taken every 30 minutes for a total of 90 minutes to determine how quickly the body metabolizes food. Some people utilize food quickly and are known as fast oxidizers. Those who use food slowly are called slow oxidizers. People are then divided into several categories, depending on whether they are acid, alkaline, or balanced blood types and whether they are fast, slow, or balanced oxidizers.

The classic lion is a fast oxidizer, acid blood type. This person feels great eating meat and other foods high in protein. Since the lion is a fast oxidizer, it needs food that is utilized by the body slowly. Fat and protein require lengthy digestion before becoming available to the body to use as an energy source. These patients require a high protein, higher fat, low carbohydrate diet, as well as various supplements and vitamins that balance the pH. Vitamin E, vitamin B-3, B-12, B-5, fish oils, zinc, iodine, and calcium will aid in this process. Items such as vitamin C in the form of ascorbic acid are very acidic and are therefore excluded.

The classic giraffe is a slow oxidizer, alkaline blood type. Because the giraffe utilizes food slowly, it needs food that is easily absorbed like fruits and vegetables. The giraffe feels best eating a vegetarian-based diet and requires less protein than the lion. Supplements to balance a giraffe's pH include alfalfa or wheat grass, vitamins and minerals like vitamin C, vitamins B-1, B-2, B-3, B-6, magnesium, chromium, and potassium may be recommended.

Metabolic Typing helps explain why some patients maintain good health eating a vegetarian diet and why others can do the same eating a high protein diet. There is no one diet that is the best for everyone. Contrary to popular belief, patients can lose weight and lower their cholesterol while consuming a diet high in protein and fat. When was the last time you saw a fat lion? Lion types have trouble with obesity and heart disease when they eat a diet high in carbohydrates. Lion types need to eat less refined carbohydrates like white bread, pasta, potatoes, and food high in sugar.

128

Opposites do attract. A lion metabolic type usually marries a giraffe metabolic type. Marion is pure giraffe. She even has the neck! She eats a vegetarian-based diet. If she eats too much fat during a meal, she has immediate bloating and feels terrible. Ross is a pure lion. A pizza will put him to sleep, but a juicy hamburger makes him feel great. Does he have a cholesterol problem? No. It is below normal.

Another aspect of determining the proper foods for a person involves checking blood type. Depending on a person's blood type, certain foods are better than others. Dr. Peter D'Adamo has written a comprehensive book on this subject titled *Eat Right for Your Type.*[2]

BLOOD TYPE

Most people know the importance of blood typing with regard to receiving a blood transfusion. It could mean the difference between life and death. Some blood types are totally incompatible. If someone with Type B blood received a blood transfusion from someone with type A blood, death could result because type B blood is incompatible with type A blood. This is because of agglutination. The type B blood agglutinates or clumps when exposed to type A blood.

Likewise, foods can cause agglutination because of the presence of lectins on their cell surfaces. Lectins are sugar-binding proteins that agglutinate or clump cells. Foods contain different lectins. Your blood type will help determine what foods may not be beneficial for you because of lectin incompatibility. This is usually the variable responsible for not being able to eat certain foods that might otherwise be considered healthy.

BODY TYPE

Another aspect of Metabolic Typing is related to Body Type. Did you ever wonder why one person gains weight around the abdomen, while others gain it in the rear end? Some people gain weight all over. There are also differences in the way people are built. Some people are "big boned" and others are twiggy. The body types not only differ in appearance, but they eat differently. For example, one body type usually loves salty foods such as chips and dip, while another type's downfall is sweets.

AUTONOMIC NERVOUS SYSTEM DOMINANCE

What about personality types? We have all heard the saying "opposites attract." One partner is a go-getter, what we might call a "type A personality," or a person with too much adrenaline. Usually a type A person is attracted to the opposite type person, so that together they balance each other. These two types are also called sympathetic dominant (lots of adrenaline) and parasympathetic dominant (lot of acetylcholine which slows the body down). This is called autonomic nervous system dominance and plays an important role in Metabolic Typing.

SUMMARY

You can now see that many different metabolic types exist. This is why one diet will not work for everyone. Caring Medical and Rehabilitation Services has developed the *Caring Medical Nutritional Analysis* which can determine the exact foods a person is to eat, depending on the results of the Metabolic Typing.* Many people are now able to quit guessing about what to eat and regain their health through Metabolic Typing.

If you would like to become a patient at Caring Medical and Rehabilitation Services and receive Metabolic Typing, please contact our office at 708-848-7789. The secretary will send you some questionnaires to complete and set you up for appointments with the doctor and in the lab for the testing. It will be important for you to come to the office after an overnight fast. The whole testing process takes about two hours.

Remember there is no one diet for everyone. Everyone requires a diet and supplement program specifically for their body type. Metabolic Typing will keep you active for life! To learn more about Metabolic Typing, read *Biobalance*, by Rudolf Wiley, Ph.D.[3]

---

* *This information has not been evaluated by the FDA, AMA, or ADA and is based on the experiences of Ross and Marion Hauser, as well as research done by Drs. Wiley, D'Adamo, and Abravanel.*

Neural Therapy

Some people experience chronic pain that is not due to ligament or tendon weakness. Some chronic pain stems from nerve irritation. This type of pain may be relieved by a treatment known as Neural Therapy.

Neural Therapy is a gentle healing technique developed in Germany that involves the injection of local anesthetics into autonomic ganglia, peripheral nerves, scars, glands, acupuncture points, trigger points, and other tissues.[1] (See Figure Appendix B-1.) What are autonomic ganglia? The body contains two nervous systems: the somatic and the autonomic. The somatic nervous system is under a person's voluntary control. The autonomic nervous system functions automatically. The autonomic ganglia is the place where the center of the autonomic nerves are located.

SOMATIC AND AUTONOMIC NERVOUS SYSTEMS

The nerves in the somatic nervous system control skin sensation and muscle movement. Picking up a cup of tea, for example, requires the somatic nervous system to sense the cup with the fingers and contract the muscles to lift the cup. These are the same nerves that are pinched in a herniated disc.

The autonomic nervous system is automatically activated. Life-sustaining functions like breathing, blood flow, pupil dilation, and perspiration are activated by the autonomic nervous system. People do not think about the blood vessels in their hands constricting when they are outside on a cold, winter day. This occurs automatically. The functioning of the autonomic nervous system is crucial as it controls blood flow throughout the body. Illness often begins when the blood flow to an extremity or an organ is decreased.

A limb with decreased blood flow feels cold and may experience dull burning pain. Even atrophy (breakdown) of the skin and muscles may occur. Decreased blood flow to an organ hinders its ability to function. Decreased blood flow to the thyroid gland may result in hypothyroidism. In this instance, the amount of thyroid hormone the body produces is decreased, resulting in sluggishness, weight gain, and lower body temperature. Does that sound like anyone you know?

Disturbed autonomic nervous system function has been implicated in the following diseases: headaches, migraines, dizziness, confusion, optic neuritis, chronic ear infections, tinnitus, vertigo, hay fever, sinusitis, tonsillitis, asthma, liver disease, gallbladder disease, menstrual pain, eczema, and a host of others.[2] Neural Therapy, because it increases blood flow, may have profoundly positive effects on such conditions.

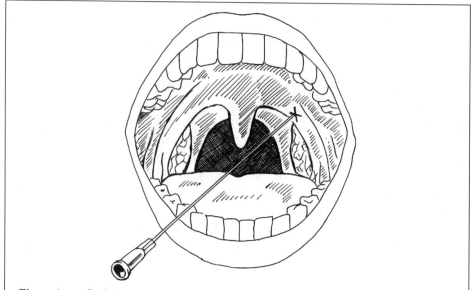

Figure Appendix B-1: Neural Therapy on the Tonsils
Any previously traumatized, surgerized or infected site or tissue can be an interference field for the autonomic nervous system.

INTERFERENCE FIELDS

The founder of Neural Therapy, Ferdinand Huneke, M.D., felt one of its beneficial effects was the elimination of interference fields. An interference field is any pathologically damaged tissue, which on account of an excessively strong or long-standing stimulus or of a summation of stimuli that cannot be abated, is in a state of unphysiological permanent excitation.[3] In layman's terms, any time a tissue is injured it can continually excite the autonomic nervous system. These centers of irritation through the autonomic nervous system may cause disease in other parts of the body.

Most interference fields are found in the head region. According to Dr. Huneke, teeth and tonsils are the two most common probably because they are close to the brain and nerves. **(See Figure Appendix B-1)** An infected tooth can set up an interference field causing a person to have chronic low back pain or a heart arrhythmia. A patient may have chronic low back pain that is unresponsive to surgical and conservative treatments because an interference field is present.

Scars are the next most common interference fields. Any scar, no matter how small or old, even if it dates back to early childhood, can be the interference field causing therapy-resistant rheumatoid arthritis, hearing loss, sciatica, or other serious disorders.[4]

A good analogy of the interference field is heart arrhythmia, or irregular heart beats. In a heart arrhythmia an area of the heart sends off an independent, electrical impulse. This impulse is not under the normal control of the heart's electrical system. It acts independently and automatically. During a heart attack, the heart may produce extra beats, called premature ventricular contractions (PVCs). One of the standard treatments for PVCs is an intravenous infusion of Lidocaine, an anesthetic. This treatment effectively stops this type of arrhythmia.

NEURAL THERAPY AS PAIN MANAGEMENT

Neural Therapy involves the injection of anesthetic solutions, such as Lidocaine or procaine, into these interference fields. The areas injected may include various areas of the teeth, tonsils, autonomic nervous system nerves, or ganglia, somatic or peripheral nerves, scars, or the area surrounding various organs. Immediate pain relief is often observed after the first injection because nerve irritation has been resolved.

Most traditional physicians are not aware of the role of the autonomic nervous system or do not diagnose problems involving it because an autonomic nervous system cannot be tested. The autonomic nervous system does not appear on x-rays; only somatic nervous system nerves can be seen.

To diagnose an autonomic nervous system problem, the clinician must understand interference fields as well as Neural Therapy. An autonomic nervous system disorder should be suspected if any of the following conditions are evident: burning pain, excessively cool or hot extremities, pale or red hands or feet, skin sensitivity to touch, scars, root canals, chronic problems occurring after an infection or accident, chronic pain not responsive to other forms of therapy, shooting burning nerve pain, pinched nerve, or a chronic medical condition that has not responded to other treatments.

While Neural Therapy is used more frequently as a healing modality in European countries than in the United States, nevertheless Caring Medical offers this treatment, if appropriate as an option after an initial consultation.

To learn more about Neural Therapy, consult the *Illustrated Atlas of the Techniques of Neural Therapy with Local Anesthetics,* a textbook from Germany.[5]

At our office, Neural Therapy has been a wonderful, adjunctive therapy for the treatment of chronic pain and illness. A person with chronic pain often has evidence of both ligament laxity and autonomic nervous system dysfunction. In such a case, both Prolotherapy and Neural Therapy are warranted. Because chronic pain sometimes has an autonomic nervous system component, many are choosing to Neural Therapy their pain away! ■

Natural Medicine Nutritional Products

Many people suffer from pain partially because their bodies have lost the ability to heal soft tissue injuries completely. If patients receive Prolotherapy for weakened ligaments or tendons, but their bodies lack vital nutrients, healing may be incomplete. It is important to consume all vital nutrients daily to assist soft tissue healing. The following are companies for nutritional products that we use in our office. They provide quality products that physicians may purchase in their offices to sell to their patients.

ORTHOMOLECULAR PRODUCTS
2771 CEDAR DRIVE
PLOVER, WI 54467
(800) 332-2351

Orthomolecular Products makes products for physicians to sell in their offices. President Gary Powers has a wide variety of high quality products. Mr. Powers is very supportive of Beulah Land Natural Medicine Clinic.

Dr. Hauser has developed several products in conjunction with Orthomolecular Products to specifically help support the connective tissues of the body:

● **OrthoProloMax:** This product has been helpful in assisting healing in all of the conditions discussed in this book, including arthritis, Fibromyalgia, sprains and strains, sports injuries, and many other chronic painful conditions. It contains MSM, Siberian Ginseng, Horsetail, RNA, Fo Ti, and the amino acids Proline and L-Cysteine, which are present in collagen.

● **Vesselmax:** This product is designed to help support the vascular connective tissue with herbs such as Gotu Kola, Horsechestnut, Butcher's Broom, and Troxerutin.

● **Cosmedix:** This product is designed to help with systemic connective tissue deficiency. This condition is characterized by a weakness in the connective tissues of the body causing a person to have such symptoms as fatigue, non-restful sleep, chronic pain, poor healing of injuries, excessive wrinkles, thinning hair, thinning skin, and brittle nails. The product has a lot of unique nutritional remedies such as Fo Ti, MSM, Biotin, PABA, Nettles Leaf, Horsetail, and a unique set of vitamins.

● **Ortho Derma:** This product will help you attain better and younger-looking skin. It contains very high dose vitamins A & D, Silica, Burdock Root, Gotu Kola, Dandelion Root, Pantothenic Acid, and other ingredients to help support the connective tissue of the skin.

● **Ortho Sports Products:** Who needs more connective tissue support than an athlete? The Ortho Sports Line is designed to help athletes build endurance and speed, while shortening the recovery time between workouts. The products contain the potent analgesics, as discussed in the MEAT protocol, such as bromelain, as well as a unique set of minerals and nutritionals designed to decrease lactic acid build-up and enhance athletic performance.

● **Ortho Lean Program For Life:** This program provides much more than weight loss products. They help speed metabolism and provide the energy so many people desperately lack. The program is designed to help increase growth hormone levels, which helps decrease fat while building muscle. The nighttime formula also has herbs to help induce deep sleep, which is necessary for soft tissue healing to occur.

KYLEA HEALTH AND NUTRITION
P.O. BOX 399
GLEN ELLYN, IL 60138
(888) 557-5700

Kylea Health and Nutrition has superb nutritional products, which are sold retail, as well as to physicians. The owner of Kylea, Joe Costello, donates 10 percent of profits to worthy charitable causes, one of them being Beulah Land.

● **Slim Trim and Stay Thin Products:** These products were developed by Ross and Marion Hauser to help enhance metabolism, provide energy, increase growth hormone levels, decrease fat, and build muscle. DayTime Metabolic Enhancer, NightTime Metabolic Enhancer, and Protein Powder are available as a package.

● **Other Products:** Kylea carries other products that are useful for general health, soft tissue healing, female conditions and others.

● We also use: **Next Level Up, CalMg, Resistance Plus, Colon Cleanse, and Energized.**

Prolotherapy Referral List

Whilst Prolotherapy is a technique that is still relatively unknown, it is gaining popularity, We have included a list of physicians whom we know personally and who utilize the Hackett-Hemwall technique of Prolotherapy daily in their practices because they regularly volunteer at Beulah Land Natural Medicine Clinic.

ROSS A. HAUSER, M.D.
CARING MEDICAL & REHABILITATION SERVICES, S.C.
715 LAKE STREET, SUITE 600
OAK PARK, ILLINOIS, 60301
708-848-7789
www.caringmedical.com
drhauser@caringmedical.com

NICOLE D. KING, M.D.
CARING WOMEN'S NATURAL HEALTH CENTER
715 LAKE STREET, SUITE 720
OAK PARK, ILLINOIS, 60301
708-848-7708
www.caringmedical.com
drhauser@caringmedical.com

RODNEY VAN PELT, M.D.
665 N. STATE ST.
UKIAH, CA 95482
707-463-1782

MARK T. WHEATON, M.D.
RIDGEHILL PROFESSIONAL BUILDING
2000 PLYMOUTH RD., SUITE 175
MINNETONKA, MN 55305
612-593-0500
drmark@wheatons.com

For further information, please see:

www.caringmedical.com

www.proloinfo.com

www.prolotherapy.com

TEACHING TAPES FOR PHYSICIANS

Teaching tapes that illustrate the technique of Prolotherapy by David Brewer, M.D., Ross Hauser, M.D., Gustav A. Hemwall, M.D., and Jean-Paul Ouellette, M.D. can be ordered by calling 708-848-7789. ∎

George S. Hackett AMA Presentations

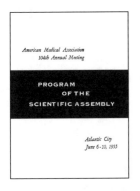

AMERICAN MEDICAL ASSOCIATION
104TH ANNUAL MEETING
PROGRAM OF THE SCIENTIFIC ASSEMBLY
ATLANTIC CITY, JUNE 6-10, 1955

DIAGNOSIS AND TREATMENT OF BACK DISABILITIES.
GEORGE S. HACKETT, CANTON, OHIO.

"Relaxation of the posterior ligaments of the spine and pelvis is the most frequent cause of back pain and disability. Diagnosis is made by trigger point pressure and confirmed by injecting an anaesthetic within the ligament. The local and referred pain are immediately reproduced and disappear within two minutes. The patient's confidence is established. Treatment consists of injection of a proliferant within the ligament which stimulates the production of bone and fibrous tissue, which becomes permanent. New areas of referred pain in the groin, buttock, and extremities have been identified during the past 16 years while making over 3,000 injections within the ligaments of 563 patients, with 82 percent considering themselves cured. Ages range from 15 to 81 years. Longest duration before treatment was 49 years; the average was 4 ½ years. X-rays of animal experiments carried out over two years reveal the proliferation of abundant permanent tissue at the fibro-osseous junction."

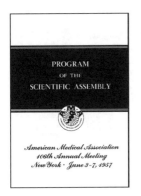

AMERICAN MEDICAL ASSOCIATION
106TH ANNUAL MEETING
PROGRAM OF THE SCIENTIFIC ASSEMBLY
NEW YORK, JUNE 3-7, 1957

PAIN, REFERRED PAIN AND SCIATICA IN
BACK DIAGNOSIS AND TREATMENT.
GEORGE S. HACKETT, MERCY HOSPITAL, CANTON, OHIO.

"Referred pain into the extremities and sciatica results more often from relaxed ligaments of unstable joints than from all other causes combined. Referred pain areas into the groin, lower abdomen, genitalia, buttock and extremities to as far as the toes from articular ligaments that support the lumbar and pelvic joints have been established from observations while making over 10,000 intraligamentous injections in the diagnosis and treatment of 1,207 patients during the past 18 years. Articular ligament relaxation has been found to be the cause of more chronic low back disability than from any other entity. The trigger points of pain of specific disabled ligaments have been established. In diagnosis, knowl-

137

edge of the referred pain areas directs attention to specific ligaments, and in conjunction with the trigger points of pain, enables the physician to accurately locate the cause of the disability. Ninety percent of the patients with joint instability are cured by the intraligamentous injection of a proliferating solution which stimulates the production of new bone and fibrous tissue cells to permanently strengthen the ligaments."

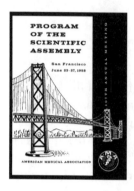

AMERICAN MEDICAL ASSOCIATION
107TH ANNUAL MEETING
PROGRAM OF THE SCIENTIFIC ASSEMBLY
SAN FRANCISCO, JUNE 23-27, 1958

CERVICAL WHIPLASH INJURY.
GEORGE S. HACKETT, CANTON, OHIO.

"Chronic whiplash cervical pain has its origin within incompetent occipital tendons and cervical articular ligaments which stretch under normal tension and permit an over-stimulation of the nonstretchable sensory nerve fibrils at the fibro-osseous junction. It results in headache and specific referred pain areas to as far as the eyes, temples, and fingers. The diagnosis is invariably confirmed by intraligamentous needling with an anesthetic solution. Eighty-two percent of 1656 patients throughout 19 years considered themselves permanently cured by Prolotherapy (rehabilitation of an incompetent structure by the proliferation of new cells—bone and fibrous tissue 'weld')."

The information in this appendix is from abstracts of Dr. Hackett's presentations and is used with permission of the American Medical Association, Chicago, Illinois. ■

Insurance Reimbursement Letters

When the issue of the efficacy of Prolotherapy found its way to the courts in Canada for the first time last year (where socialized medicine reigns and governmental bodies do not want to pay for certain medical procedures) for lumbar disc syndrome, the verdict read "on the basis of all the evidence, the Prolotherapy treatment administered to the patient was and is a safe and efficacious treatment." [1]

Similar cases have been noted in the United States. When an insurer in the state of Washington did not pay for the Prolotherapy treatment that relieved a person's chronic low back pain, the case was brought to trial. The Washington State Health Care Authority found that the Sclerotherapy (Prolotherapy) treatments the patient received for back pain were "medically necessary."

The Washington State Heath Care Authority also ruled that the treatments needed to be paid by the insurer. This judgement was made June 8, 1992 by Margaret T. Stanley, Administrator, Washington State Health Care, in the case of Joel M. Greene vs. Uniform Medical Plan. [2]

In the following pages, copies of letters from the Chicago Medical Society (one of the largest branches of the American Medical Association) and insurance carriers regarding reimbursement for Prolotherapy are provided. Please note on three separate occasions, the Medical Practice Committee of the Chicago Medical Society found Prolotherapy to be an accepted procedure that deserved reimbursement by the insurance carrier.

Realize that insurance companies hold the right whether or not to reimburse for a specific therapy. The attached letters are for individual patients and reimbursement decisions were made on a case by case basis. All names and personal information have been withheld to respect the privacy of the individuals. ∎

Chicago
Medical Society
The Medical Society of Cook County

310 SOUTH MICHIGAN AVENUE, CHICAGO, ILLINOIS 60604. TELEPHONE (312) 922-0417

April 20, 1976

Gustav Hemwall, M.D.
715 Lake Street
Oak Park, IL 60301

> Re:
> Carrier: Aetna Life & Casualty
> Date of Treatment: August 10, 1975
> CMS No. 76-M-005

Dear Doctor Hemwall:

In response to the insurance carrier's request of whether your
treatment is an approved and appropriate method, the Subcommittee
on Insurance Mediation has made a decision on the above entitled
matter.

On the basis of the information presented, it the Committee's
opinion that this procedure is an accepted procedure.

By copy of this letter, the insurance carrier will be informed of
our recommendation.

Cordially,

Carell Hutchinson, JR., M.D.
Chairman
Subcommittee on Insurance Mediation

CH:scm
cc: Aetna Life & Casualty

Chicago
Medical Society
The Medical Society of Cook County

515 NORTH DEARBORN STREET, CHICAGO, ILLINOIS 60610. TELEPHONE (312) 670-2550

November 5, 1987

RE: Prolotherapy
Chubb Life America Insurance Co.
Renate Stollenwerk/patient
Group Policy No. 314295
Claim No. 725514

Dear

We apologize for the length of time this review has taken, however the Medical Practice Committee of the Chicago Medical Society has spent much time reviewing the subject of Prolotherapy. Attached is a copy of an article published in The Western Journal of Medicine, 1982, which is a study that attempts to establish the value of Prolotherapy. In addition, we have enclosed a list of references that address the use of this procedure.

The term Prolotherapy has not found favor with many insurance companies because it does not fit with their various codes. However, upon reviewing a list of procedures that have HCFA assigned codes published by Blue Shield of Illinois (HCSC) 5/15/86, Prolotherapy is coded M0076 on page 84. It is our understanding that two years ago, the Prolotherapy Association was incorporated into a new organization called the American Association of Orthopaedic Medicine. The insurance company may wish to contact this association for additional scientific studies.

We understand that this procedure has been used by many medical and osteopathic physicians both in this country and in Europe. It is significant that Dr. Hemwall has performed this procedure on many people for almost 30 years and our Society has never received a complaint on the use of the procedure. It appears to the committee that this record speaks for successful treatment, and it is long past the stage where it is considered experimental. It is our opinion that an insurance carrier is not in a position to declare a method that is not widely used, but apparently successful, an improper one.

In light of our current review, it is the opinion of the Medical Practice Committee that the procedure of ligament injection, known as Prolotherapy, is a clinically accepted procedure and we recommend payment of the physicians fees by the insurance company.

We thank you for bringing your concerns to our attention and by copy of this letter and attached materials, Chubb LifeAmerica Insurance Company will be informed of our recommendation.

Sincerely,

Peter C. Pulos, M.D.
Chairman
Medical Practice Committee

PCP:lm
cc: Steven Prylak
Assistant Vice President
Group Claims Department
Chubb LifeAmerica

encls.

Chicago
Medical Society
The Medical Society of Cook County

810 SOUTH MICHIGAN AVENUE, CHICAGO, ILLINOIS 60604. TELEPHONE (312) 922-0417

November 1, 1979

Miss Karen M. Heckinger
Legal Research Assistant
Life Investors Insurance
   Company of America.
814 Commerce Drive
Oak Brook, IL   60521

Re: CMS File 79-G-069

Your File
   Policy No. F-9-3888
   National Ass'n. Business Owners

Dear Miss Heckinger:

After extensive inquiries by the Medical Practice Committee on the efficacy and the legitimacy of the treatment referred to as 'prolotherapy' we are left with the conclusion that there is no body of scientific data which supports this method of medical treatment. While we are unable to state that the treament is effective and accepted by the medical community, neither can we state that it is rejected by the medical community since we do not have scientific data upon which to base our judgment.

It is the opinion of the Committee that, while the treatment does not enjoy widespread acceptance in medical circles, it is a well recognized procedure in veterinary medicine: animal models of disease and treatment form the basis for a great deal of medical knowledge and progress.

It is significant to this Committee that Dr. Hemwall has performed this procedure on a great many people over an eighteen year period of time and our Society has never received a patient complaint on the procedure. It appears to us that this record speaks for successful treatment. We do not feel that either we, or an insurance carrier, are in a position to declare an uncommon, but apparently successful, procedure as an improper one. Because the method is not widely used does not mean that it is not compensable.

A search of our records reveals that another Committee of our Society was presented with a similar question regarding 'prolotherapy' and they found it an accepted procedure and recommend-ed payment of the physician's fees. We agree.

Sincerely,

Michael Treister, Dr. D
Michael Treister, M.D.
Chairman
Medical Practice Committee

MT:WDF/SFO:vvm

xc: Gustav A. Hemwall, M.D.
    Edward J. King, Counsel

142

CENTRAL STATES
SOUTHEAST AND
SOUTHWEST AREAS
HEALTH AND WELFARE FUND

9377 W Higgins Rd
Rosemont IL 60018-4938
(800) 323-5000

April 23, 1996

ROSS A HAUSER MD
715 LAKE ST SUITE 600
OAK PARK   IL 60301

RE:

Dear Dr. Hauser :

This letter is in reply to your recent inquiry regarding
need for prolotherapy treatments.

I am happy to say that the prolotherapy treatments will be payable
for four sessions one month apart from each other under the Major
Medical portion of Benefit Plan ET1. Under this Plan, there is a
$100 per calendar year deductible ($200 for the family). Once that
has been met, we will pay 80% of our reasonable and customary
allowance for all remaining eligible charges.   must be
covered on the date(s) on which services are rendered.

If you have any questions, please write the Research and
Correspondence Department at P.O. Box 5111, Des Plaines, IL 60017.

Sincerely,

Aileen M. Troia
Analyst
Research & Correspondence Dept.

cc:
cc: Local Union No. 706

M M A

Mennonite Mutual Aid
1110 North Main Street
Post Office Box 483
Goshen, IN 46527

Toll-free: 1-800-348-7468
Telephone: 219 533-9511
Fax: 219 533-5264

June 17, 1997

Ross A. Hauser, M.D.
Caring Medical & Rehab Services, Inc.
715 Lake Street, Ste 600
Oak Park, IL 60301

Insured:
Patient: Agreement No.: 5090476
Effective Date: February 1, 1990

Thank you for inquiring about   's benefits for Prolotherapy. Our
medical review team has reviewed the packet of information you sent.

We will approve coverage for up to three treatments. After the $1,000 is
met, we will pay 80 percent of the next $5,000, then 100 percent to the end
of the calendar year. The maximum lifetime benefit is $1 million. The
deductible and coinsurance are applied each calendar year.

Benefits are limited to the reasonable and customary charges and the medical
team will review for proper coding.

A final decision on any claim cannot be made until we receive the actual
charges and review them according to the guidelines of the certificate.

Thank you for contacting us to verify the benefits. If you have further
questions about coverage we provide, please let me know.

Sincerely,

Polly Kauffman
Polly Kauffman
Managed Care Assistant

cc:

Beulah Land Natural Medicine Clinic

Beulah Land Natural Medicine Clinic is a free clinic devoted through the grace of God to the prevention and treatment of human disease. This is accomplished through prayer, faithfulness to God through Jesus Christ, rest, nutrition, exercise, and the utilization of natural substances for healing and wellness.

Beulah Land Natural Medicine Clinic is located in very rural southern Illinois in the town of Thebes. Thebes is located one hour north of Paducah, Kentucky; one hour south of Carbondale, Illinois; and 30 minutes west of Cape Girardeau, Missouri. We started the clinic in 1994.

Why would a Chicago couple choose Thebes, Illinois to start a charity natural medicine clinic? Good question. In 1985, we each dedicated our lives to what we felt and continue to feel is the most important thing in life: faith in God through Jesus Christ. We both realized that where we go after this earthly life is the most important factor in our beliefs. The things of this world are finite; eternity lasts forever.

We both came to realize that what the Bible said was true. The Bible speaks about heaven in Revelation 21:27 saying, "Nothing impure will ever enter into it, nor will anyone who does what shameful or deceitful, but only those whose names are written in the Lamb's book of life." [1] We wanted to have eternal life with God. We wanted to see our names written in the Lamb's book of life.

We realized that in order to have eternal life with God in heaven, we must accept Jesus Christ as our Savior. Our own works or accomplishments could not cleanse the impurities (sins) in our lives. The only way this could happen was to accept the sacrifice of Jesus Christ for our sins and to believe that He died and rose again. We both did this. For this reason, we believe that our names are written in the Lamb's book of life.

Shortly after this experience, we joined Harrison Street Bible Church in Oak Park, Illinois. The church's senior pastor and his wife, John and Louisa Blakemore, were originally from Olive Branch, a small town in southern Illinois. Pastor John had a special place in his heart for the people of this area, even though he was working in Oak Park.

Pastor John's son, Peter, returned to Oak Park to co-pastor Harrison Street Bible Church after receiving theological training at Bob Jones University. Pastor Peter and his family soon became some of our closest friends and confidants. Pastor Peter was the kindest man we have ever known. Under his encouragement, we started a charity natural medicine clinic at Harrison Street Bible Church in 1991. This clinic met in the church basement and was staffed by volunteers.

In early 1994, we decided we needed a weekend away from our usual routine. What could be farther away than Thebes, Illinois, which is a mere 400 miles away from Chicago and located out in the middle of the country? We got much more than we bargained for by the end of the trip. We ended up buying a 120-acre piece of property surrounded by a national forest on three sides. We named the property after Pastor John's favorite song: "Beulah Land." Beulah Land comes from the Bible verse Isaiah 62:4: "No longer will they call you Deserted, or name your land Desolate. But you will be called Hephzibah, and your land Beulah; for the LORD will take delight in you, and your land will be married."

This verse describes the restoration of the relationship between God and His people Israel. We felt that this land would be restored, just as Israel had been restored. There is now a house on the property where all of the volunteers reside during the clinic days.

In late 1994, the first Beulah Land Natural Medicine Clinic was held in the basement of the First Baptist Church in Thebes, Illinois. The clinic offers many state of the art natural medicine techniques including nutritional counseling, natural hormone treatments, chiropractic manipulation, physiotherapy, Metabolic Typing, intravenous therapies, and, of course, Prolotherapy. Volunteers from all over the United States staff the Beulah Land Natural Medicine Clinic. The doctors who regularly volunteer with us are Kurt Ehling, D.C., a wonderful chiropractic physician from Morton, Illinois; Rodney Van Pelt, M.D., an expert in Prolotherapy from Ukiah, California; Mark Wheaton, M.D, another expert in Prolotherapy from Minnetonka, Minnesota; and William Hambach, D.C., a very skilled chiropractor from Oak Park, Illinois

The clinic is an outreach ministry to help people in the same manner as Jesus did. Many people sought help from Jesus for physical illnesses. This is well illustrated in the Bible verse Matthew 4:23: "Jesus went throughout Galilee, teaching in the synagogues, preaching the good news of the kingdom, and healing every disease and sickness among the people."[2] He often gave them encouragement to live justly and uprightly and for people to commit their ways to God. We try to do just that at Beulah Land Natural Medicine Clinic.

We hope that Beulah Land Natural Medicine Clinic will become a renowned medical center like the Mayo Clinic—except that natural medicine would be practiced and the people would receive the best treatments free of charge. Due to the devastating effects of chronic illnesses, many people do not have the financial resources to receive natural medicine therapies. Beulah Land is a place where treatments are offered free of charge and hope is given.

Since 1994, Beulah Land Ministries has been formed as a not-for-profit, tax-exempt corporation that runs Beulah Land Natural Medicine Clinic. We see more and more patients at each clinic. We are very close to outgrowing our current space at the First Baptist Church. We hope to be able to build a facility in the near future where care can be provided year-round. We look forward to what God has in store for us in the future.

Beulah Land Ministries can always use additional assistance. If you are interested in volunteering to work in the clinic or to help with the building project, please let us know. If you feel lead to make a tax-deductible donation, please contact us!

TO CONTACT BEULAH LAND NATURAL MEDICINE CLINIC:
Write to:
Beulah Land • RR1 Box 189,Thebes, IL 62990 • 708-802-1453 (Voice Mail)
URL: www.beulahlandinfo.com
E-Mail: beulamed@midwest.net

OR CONTACT OUR OAK PARK OFFICE AT:
Caring Medical and Rehabilitation Services
715 Lake St., Suite 600 • Oak Park, IL 60301
URL: www.caringmedical.com
E-Mail: drhauser@caringmedical.com

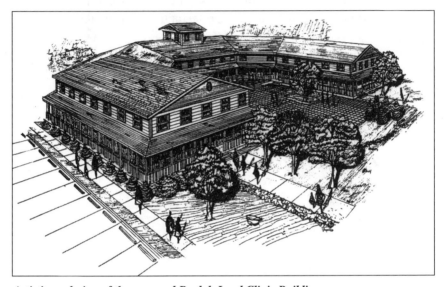

Artist's rendering of the proposed Beulah Land Clinic Building

Please consider a tax-deductible donation to Beulah Land Natural Medicine Clinic. Your gift of any amount will help those less fortunate to get the medical attention they need! You can make your donations many ways!

BY CHECK:
Mail to: Beulah Land Ministries ℅ Caring Medical and Rehabilitation Services • 715 Lake St., Suite 600 Oak Park, IL 60301

BY CREDIT CARD:
Call: 708-848-7789

Letters of Appreciation

Because of the success of Prolotherapy in relieving pain, we have quite a collection of thank you letters from all over the country and around the world, from patients and doctors who have learned this technique. We enjoy receiving these letters. Believe it or not, seldom do physicians hear the words "thank you." These are words that we all need to say more often.

We would like to take this opportunity to say thank you to the patients that have had enough confidence in us to utilize the technique of Prolotherapy to relieve their pain.

We hope you enjoy these thank you letters that have been an encouragement to us. We hope some day to receive a thank you letter from you when you Prolo your pain away! ■

Marion A Hauser, MS, RD
Ross A. Hauser M.D.

Ross and Marion Hauser

Ross A. Hauser, M.D.
Caring Medical & Rehabilitation Services, S.C.
715 Lake Street, Suite 600
Oak Park, Illinois, 60301
September 16, 1998

Dear Dr. Hauser:

Since I first heard of you in 1995, and later while working by your side for two years, I recognized you as a skilled doctor. Now I have had the excellent experience of living with and caring for one of the patients you have helped with your treatment of Prolotherapy.

This patient, Dr. Wallace Erickson, had been taking Darvocet most of the six months I have been with him. When his internist took him off this narcotic, the only options he gave Dr. Erickson for dealing with his chronic back and hip pain was to increase his Advil dosage to 16 capsules per day or undergo a highly controversial surgery of cutting some nerves in the spinal column. Taking the conservative approach and 16 Advil did very little to improve Dr. E's condition or quality of life. Pain debilitated him. Dr. Erickson lost his motivation to be involved with life, including daily personal care. He spent his days between the couch and the bed, searching for relief from his agony.

Since he had his first Prolotherapy treatment from you on September 3, 1998, very little has stopped him! The afternoon of the treatment he spent six hours out with his children, enjoying a circus and dinner (sitting the whole time), activities that would have been unthinkable in the past. Since then, he has had the energy and motivation to go out almost daily. Before Prolotherapy, encouraging him to walk or go out was like 'pulling teeth,' but now he is the initiator of such activities!! He still has occasional times of pain, but his good times are more frequent and of longer duration. He has been more alert and talkative, regaining his sense of humor and curiosity for life.

Thank you!! Thank you so much for helping restore quality of life to a man who has so much living ahead of him! I realize God is the Miracle Worker, but He has used you and the incredible technique of Prolotherapy as His tool!

Sincerely,

Alta S. Mo

Alta Morris
Care-giver to Dr. Wallace Erickson and former co-worker with Dr. Hauser

February 28, 1999

Dear Dr. Houser,

I just wanted to drop you a note and tell you about the part Prolo Therapy has had in my life.

In 1971, shortly after I got married I ruptured my first disk doing exercises. I had my first back surgery.

In 1976 I had my second surgery on the second ruptured disk. And again in 1977 I had my third surgery. After the third surgery my orthopedic surgeon told me he removed a massive amount of scar tissue. He said my back would always be weak and probably need other surgeries in the future. He only gave me a fifty percent chance of living a normal active life and being able to work until retirement age.

Two months after my third surgery a friend told me about Dr. Hemwall and Prolo Therapy. I called Dr. Hemwall and set up an appointment. Dr. Hemwall treated me and told me to rest for a few weeks and then go back to work.

For eighteen years I played softball, hiked, and lived an active life. At age 45 I learned how to downhill ski and have done so for 10 years.

At age 51 I ruptured another disk. In 1995 and 1996 I had my fourth and fifth surgery because of extreme ruptures. After recovery I once again sought out Prolo Therapy for help.

In 1996 I retired after working for 30 years in the same company. I love being retired. I will turn 56 in April of this year. I walk four miles, three times a week, and swim 50 laps in the pool at the health club, three days a week.

I just wanted to say thank you for being in Chicago. I trust you and your staff and especially Prolo Therapy. I have no fear about recommending you and the treatment to my friends, either.

Sincerely,

Richard D. Nesseth

Richard D. Nesseth

February 19, 1997

RECEIVED MAR 1 0 1997

Dr. Ross Hauser
Caring Medical & Rehabilitation Service, S.C.
715 Lake Street, Suite 600
Oak Park, Illinois 60301
Tel (708) 848-7789   REF:DRRUSS.WPS

Dear Dr. Ross Hauser:

First I would like to say may God bless you and your wife for the wonderful work that you do for the Lord!
I would like to give my personal testimony of how God used you, and the medicine that you gave me to cure me of back pain.

I had low back pain for more than eight years. Through I visited many doctors here in Mexico, no one had a definitive cure for my problem. Throughout this time I took several medicine- they were just to control the pain. They did not help the problem.

I am really grateful that a brother in Christ that work for the Institute of Basic Principles gave me your name, address and phone number so I could visit you in Chicago. My diagnosis is Lumbar Scoliosis. Last August 1996 in Chicago I received my first prolotherapy treatment of forthy injections. My second treatment was in Mexico City December 1996, I received twenty injections there. Now I do not have any pain at all. Finally I can rest at night and have a normal life without pain. In January 1997, Dr. Gerardo Cajero also injected my kness for pain that I was having in them.

The Lord has blessed us a lot here in Mexico. Dr. Cajero has many patients in Mexico City and in Monterrey. The mexican people are really grateful to you because you invest your time in training Dr. Cajero.

Also we are really interested in any information that you might have on conferences or medical literature to support this treatment, which we can present to the Mexican Medical Asociation. Dr. Cajero is very interested in forming a Society of Prolotherapy here in Mexico. Please pray about that.

Again, thank you so much for your help and for willingness to serve the Lord and others.

With Love,

Miriam Morales

June 16, 1997

Dear Dr. Hauser,

First I would like to thank you for bringing your Clinic to Southern Illinois.

I was diagnosed with Osteoarthritis in both knees and lower back last year. I was in severe pain and almost to the point of not being able to walk or do simple household tasks. The Specialist had told me I would have to have my right knee replaced or I would probably not be able to walk without severe pain. So I was almost willing to try anything. I went to the Beulah Land Clinic in Thebes at the suggestion of a friend and am very glad I did. I had Prolotherapy on both knees and lower back. I have had three treatments so far and am virtually pain free in my left knee and lower back. I still have some pain in my right knee, but not even a quarter of what it used to be. I am back to walking any where from three to five miles a day, so feel very fortunate. I would highly recommend this treatment to any one who has a problem like mine.

Again Thank-You very much and am looking forward to your return trip to Southern Illinois

Yours Truly,
Sharon Calvert

March 22, 1999

Caring Medical & Rehabilitation Services, S.C.
715 Lake Street, Suite 600
Oak Park, Illinois 60301

Dear Dr. Hauser:

I have been ecstatic about the results I received from ONE prolotherapy treatment several months ago. I am 31 years old and have suffered with Fibromyalgia for 12 years.

I had a car accident that I was not able to recover from. Attempts to find permanent relief from acupuncture, chiropractic, physical therapy, pain medications and nutritional supplements were unsatisfactory. Even though many doctors maintain Fibromyalgia pain can be relieved by exercise, I still had pain with regular exercise.

Previously, I suffered from incapacitating burning sensations in trigger points, limited range of motion, lack of energy, stiffness and severe headaches. After doing extensive reading on prolotherapy, I was confident that I had to try it. I was expected to have several treatments. However, after the first session I was given a test that simulated pain. That test revealed normal levels of pain! I was released from prolotherapy! I have continued to only take the nutritional supplements Dr. Hauser recommended; and, I have avoided any anti-inflammatory medications.

I can't even express the thrill of regaining hope to live a life without pain. Prior to prolotherapy, I had resigned myself to just "cope" with the pain and to adjust my life to the pain. That is how so many doctors tell patients to deal with chronic pain. I am so grateful that Dr. Hauser is proactively making a difference to rid our lives of pain!

Sincerely,

Kari L. Fair

Kari L. Fair

DEDICATION
1. *The Holy Bible*, New International Version, 1 Cor. 11:1

ACKNOWLEDGEMENTS
1.. *The Holy Bible*, New International Version, Psalm 71:14-16.

CHAPTER 2
THE TECHNIQUE AND ITS HISTORY

1. Schneider, R. Fatality after injection of sclerosing agent to precipitate fibro-osseous proliferation. Journal of the American Medical Association. 1959; 170:1768-1772.
2. An abstract of a poster presentation (poster #49) at the 59th Annual Assembly of the American Academy of Physical Medicine and Rehabilitation printed in the Archives of Physical Medicine and Rehabilitation.
3. Kim, M. Myofascial trigger point therapy: comparison of dextrose, water, saline, and lidocaine. *Archives of Physical Medicine and Rehabilitation.* 1997; 78:1028.
4. Klein, R. A randomized double-blind trial of dextrose-glycerine-phenol injections for chronic, low back pain. *Journal of Spinal Disorders.* 1993; 6:23-33.
5. Ongley, M. A new approach to the treatment of chronic low back pain. *Lancet.* 1987; 2:143-146.
6. Travell, J. *Myofascial Pain and Dysfunction.* Baltimore, MD: Williams and Wilkins, 1983, pp. 103-164.
7. Wiesel, S. A study of computer-related assisted tomography. The incidence of positive CAT scans in an asymptomatic group of patients. *Spine.* 1984; 9:549-551.
8. From a phone conversation with C. Everett Koop, M.D., on May 16, 1997.
9. Boyd, Nathaniel. *Stay Out of the Hospital.* New York, NY: The Two Continents Publishing Group, Ltd., 1976, pp. 125-128.
10. Ibid.

CHAPTER 3
WHY PROLOTHERAPY WORKS

1. Hackett, G. *Ligament and Tendon Relaxation Treated by Prolotherapy.* Third Edition. Springfield, IL: Charles C. Thomas Publisher, 1958, p. 5.
2. Babcock, P. et al. *Webster's Third New International Dictionary.* Springfield, MA: G.& C. Merriam Co., 1971, p. 1815.
3. Browner, B. *Skeletal Trauma.* Volume 1. Philadelphia, PA: W.B. Saunders Company, 1992, pp. 87-88.

4. Deese, J. Compressive neuropathies of the lower extremity. *The Journal of Musculoskeletal Medicine.* 1988; November: 68-91.

5. Kayfetz, D. Occipital-cervical (whiplash) injuries treated by prolotherapy. *Medical Trail Technique Quarterly.* 1963; June: 9-29

6. Rhalmi, S. Immunohistochemical study of nerves in lumbar spine ligaments. *Spine.* 1993; 18:264-267.

7. Ahmed, M. Neuropeptide Y, tyrosine hydroxylase and vasoactive intestinal polypeptide immunoreactive nerve fibers in the vertebral bodies, discs, dura mater, and spinal ligaments of the rat lumbar spine. *Spine.* 1993; 18:268-273.

8. Hackett G., Hemwall, G., and Montgomery, G. *Ligament and Tendon Relaxation Treated by Prolotherapy.* Fifth Edition. Oak Park, IL: Gustav A. Hemwall, Publisher, 1993, p. 20.

9. Rhalmi, S. Immunohistochemical study of nerves in lumbar spine ligaments. *Spine.* 1993; 18:264-267.

10. Ahmed, M. Neuropeptide Y, tyrosine hydroxylase and vasoactive intestinal polypeptide-immunoreactive nerve fibers in the vertebral bodies, discs, dura mater, and spinal ligaments of the rat lumbar spine. *Spine.* 1993; 18:268-273.

11. Robbins, S. *Pathologic Basis of Disease.* Third Edition. Philadelphia, PA: W.B. Saunders Co., 1984, p. 40.

CHAPTER 4
PROLOTHERAPY PROVIDES RESULTS

1. Hackett, G. *Ligament and Tendon Relaxation Treated by Prolotherapy.* Third Edition. Springfield, IL: Charles C. Thomas Publisher, 1958, p. 5 and Hackett, G. Low back pain. *The British Journal of Physical Medicine.* 1956; 19:25-33.

2. Hackett, G. Referred pain and sciatica in diagnosis of low back disability *Journal of the American Medical Association.* 1957; 163:183-185.

3. Hackett, G. Joint stabilization. *American Journal of Surgery.* 1955; 89:968-973.

4. Hackett, G. Referred pain from low back ligament disability. *AMA Archives of Surgery.* 73:878-883, November 1956.

5. Liu, Y. An in situ study of the influence of a sclerosing solution in rabbit medial collateral ligaments and its junction strength. *Connective Tissue Research.* 1983; 2:95-102.

6. Maynard, J. Morphological and biomechanical effects of sodium morrhuate on tendons. *Journal of Orthopaedic Research.* 1985; 3:236-248.

7. Ibid.

8. Klein, R. Proliferant injections for low back pain: histologic changes of injected ligaments and objective measures of lumbar spine mobility before and after treatment. *Journal of Neurology, Orthopedic Medicine and Surgery.* 1989; 10:141-144.

9. Interview with Thomas Dorman, M.D. *Nutrition & Healing.* 1994; pp. 5-6.

10. Dorman, T. Treatment for spinal pain arising in ligaments using prolotherapy: A retrospective study. *Journal of Orthopaedic Medicine.* 1991; 13(1):13-19.

11. Ongley, M. and Dorman T. et al. Ligament instability of knees: A new approach to treatment. *Manual Medicine.* 1988; 3:152-154.

12. Klein R. A randomized double-blind trial of dextrose-glycerine-phenol injections for chronic, low back pain. *Journal of Spinal Disorders.* 1993; 6:23-33.

13. Ongley, M. A new approach to the treatment of chronic low back pain. *Lancet.* 1987; 2:143-146.

14. Schwartz, R. Prolotherapy: A literature review and retrospective study. *Journal of Neurology, Orthopedic Medicine, and Surgery.* 1991;12:220-223.

15. Wilkinson, H. Broad spectrum approach to the failed back. Lecture presentation at the American College of Osteopathic Pain Management and Sclerotherapy meeting on May 3, 1997.

CHAPTER 5
ANSWERS TO COMMON QUESTIONS ABOUT PROLOTHERAPY

1. Meyers, A. *Prolotherapy treatment of low back pain and sciatica.* Bulletin of the Hospital for Joint Disease. 1961; 22:1.

2. Woo, S. Injury and repair of the musculoskeletal soft tissues. American Academy of Orthopedic Surgeons. 1987.

3. Mankin, H. Localization of tritiated thymidine in articular cartilage of rabbits inhibits growth in immature cartilage. *Journal of Bone & Joint Surgery.* 1962; 44A:682.

4. Butler, D. Biomechanics of ligaments and tendons. *Exercise and Sports Scientific Review.* 1975; 6:125.

5. Bland, J. *Disorders of the Cervical Spine.* Philadelphia, PA: W.B. Saunders, 1987.

6. Letter written April 20, 1976 by Carell Hutchingson, Jr., M.D., as chairman of the Subcommittee on Insurance Mediation for the Chicago Medical Society, CMS No. 76-M-005.

7. Letter written November 1, 1979 by Michael Treister, M.D., as chairman of the Medical Practice Committee for the Chicago Medical Society regarding CMS File 79-G-069.

8. Letter written November 5, 1987 by Peter C. Pulos, M.D., as chairman of the Medical Practice Committee for the Chicago Medical Society regarding Claim No. 725514.

9. Reeves, K. *Technique of Prolotherapy.* From Physiatric Procedures in Clinical Practice. Philadelphia, PA: Hanley and Belfus, Inc., 1994, pp. 57-70.

10. Reeves, K. Prolotherapy, present and future applications in soft-tissue pain and disability. *Physical Medicine and Rehabilitation Clinics of North America.* 1995; 6:917-925.

11. Dorman, T. *Diagnosis and Injection Techniques in Orthopedic Medicine.* Baltimore, MD: Williams and Wilkins, 1991.

12. Faber, W., and Walker, M. Instant pain relief. Milwaukee, WI: *Biological Publications,* 1991.

13. Faber, W., and Walker, M. *Pain, Pain Go Away.* San Jose, CA: ISHI Press International, 1990.

14. Butler, D. Biomechanics of ligaments and tendons. *Exercise & Sports Scientific Review.* 1975; 6:125.

15. Tipton, C. Influence of immobilization, training, exogenous hormones, and surgical repair of knee ligaments from hypophysectomized rats. *American Journal of Physiology.* 1971; 221:1114.

16. Nachemson, A. Some mechanical properties of the third human lumbar interlaminar ligament. *Journal of Biomechanics.* 1968; 1:211.

17. Akeson, W. The Connective Tissue Response to Immobility: An Accelerated Aging Response. *Experimental Gerontology.* 1968; 3:239.

18. Travell, J. *Myofascial Pain and Dysfunction.* Baltimore, MD: Williams and Wilkins, 1983, pp. 103-164.

19. Schumacher, H. *Primer on the Rheumatic Diseases.* Tenth Edition. Atlanta, GA: Arthritis Foundation, 1993, pp. 8-11.

20. Ballard, W. Biochemical aspects of aging and degeneration in the invertebral disc.*Contemporary Orthopaedics.* 1992; 24:453-458.

21. Jacobs, R. Pathogenesis of idiopathic scoliosis. Chicago, IL: *Scoliosis Research Society,* 1984, pp. 107-118.

22. Crowninsheild, R. The strength and failure characteristics of rat medial collateral ligaments. *Journal of Trauma.* 1976; 16:99.

23. Travell, J. *Myofascial Pain and Dysfunction.* Baltimore, MD: Williams and Wilkins, 1983, pp. 103-164.

24. Tipton, C. Response of adrenalectomized rats to exercise. *Endocrinology.* 1972; 91:573.

25. Tipton, C. Response of thyroidectomized rats to training*American Journal of Physiology.* 1972; 215:1137.

26. Bucci, L. *Nutrition Applied to Injury Rehabilitation and Sports Medicine.* Boca Raton, FL: CRC Press, 1995, pp. 167-176.

27. Batmanghelidj, F. *Your Body's Many Cries for Water.* Second Edition. Falls Church, VA: Global Health Solutions, Inc., 1996, pp. 8-11.

28. Welbourne, T. Increased plasma bicarbonate and growth hormone after an oral glutamine load. *American Journal of Clinical Nutrition.* 1995; pp. 1058-1061.

29. Hurson, M. Metabolic effects of arginine in a healthy elderly population. *Journal of Parenteral and Enteral Nutrition.* 1995; pp. 227-230.

30. Dominguez, R. and Gajda, R. Total body training. East Dundee, IL: *Moving Force Systems,* 1982, pp. 33-37.

31. Laros, G. Influence of physical activity on ligament insertions in the knees of dogs. *Journal of Bone and Joint Surgery* (Am). 1971; 53:275.

32. Hunter, L. *Rehabilitation of the Injured Knee.* St. Louis, MO: The C.V. Mosby Company, 1984.

33. Arnoczky, S. Meniscal degeneration due to knee instability: an experimental study in the dog. *Trans. Orthop. Res. Soc.* 1979; 4:79.

34. Hunter, L. *Rehabilitation of the Injured Knee.* St. Louis, MO: The C.V. Mosby Company, 1984.

35. Arnoczky, S. Meniscal degeneration due to knee instability: an experimental study in the dog. *Trans. Orthop. Res. Soc.* 1979; 4:79.

36. Tipton, C. The influence of physical activity on ligaments and tendons. *Med. Sci. Sports.* 1975; 7:165.

37. Woo, S. Effect of immobilization and exercise on strength characteristics of bone-medial collateral ligament-bone complex. *Am. Soc. Mech. Eng. Symp.* 1979; 32:62.

38. Hunter, L. *Rehabilitation of the Injured Knee.* St. Louis, MO: The C.V. Mosby Company, 1984.

39. Noyes, F. Biomechanics of anterior cruciate ligament failure: an analysis of strain rate sensitivity and mechanism of failure in primates. *Journal of Bone & Joint Surgery.* 1974; 56A:236.

40. Noyes, F. Biomechanics of ligament failure: an analysis of immobilization, exercise and reconditioning effects in primates. *Journal of Bone & Joint Surgery.* 1974; 56A:1406.

41. Laros, G. Influence of physical activity on ligament insertions in the knees of dogs. *Journal of Bone & Joint Surgery* (Am). 1971; 53A:275.

42. Hunter, L. *Rehabilitation of the Injured Knee.* St. Louis, MO: The C.V. Mosby Company, 1984.

43. Akeson, W. Immobility effects on synovial joints: The pathomechanics of joint contracture. *Biorheology.* 1980; 17:95.

44. Ho, S. Comparison of various icing times in decreasing bone metabolism and blood flow in the knee. *The American Journal of Sports Medicine.* 1990; 18:376-378.

45. McGaw, W. The effect of tension on collagen remodeling by fibroblasts: a sterological ultrastructural study. *Connective Tissue Research.* 1986; 14:229-235.

46. Bucci, L. *Nutrition Applied to Injury Rehabilitation and Sports Medicine.* Boca Raton, FL: CRC Press, 1995, pp. 167-176.

47. Hardy, M. The biology of scar formation. *Physical Therapy.* 1989; 69:12.

48. Mishra, D. Anti-inflammatory medication after muscle injury: A treatment resulting in short-term improvement but subsequent loss of muscle function. *Journal of Bone & Joint Surgery.* 1995; 77A:1510-1519.

49. Brandt, K. Should osteoarthritis be treated with nonsteroidal anti-inflammatory drugs? *Rheumatic Disease Clinics of North America.* 1993; 19:697-712.

50. Brandt, K. The effects of salicylates and other nonsteroidal anti-inflammatory drugs on articular cartilage. *American Journal of Medicine.* 1984; 77:65-69.

51. Obeid, G. Effect of Ibuprofen on the healing and remodeling of bone and articular cartilage in the rabbit temporomandibular joint. *Journal of Oral and Maxillofacial Surgeons.* 1992; pp. 843-850.

52. Dupont, M. The efficacy of anti-inflammatory medication in the treatment of the acutely sprained ankle. *The American Journal of Sports Medicine.* 1987; 15:41-45.

53. Newman, N. Acetabular bone destruction related to nonsteroidal anti-inflammatory drugs. *The Lancet.* 1985; July 6:11-13.

54. Serup, J. and Oveson, J. Salicylate arthropathy: accelerated coxarthrosis during long-term treatment with acetyl salicylic acid. *Praxis.* 1981; 70:359.

55. Ronningen, H. and Langeland, N. Indomethacin treatment in osteoarthritis of the hip joint. *Acta Orthopedica Scandanavia.* 1979; 50:169-174.

56. Newman, N. Acetabular bone destruction related to nonsteroidal anti-inflammatory drugs. *The Lancet.* 1985; July 6:11-13.

57. Serup, J. and Ovesen, J. Salicylate arthropathy: accelerated coxarthrosis during long-term treatment with acetyl salicylic acid. *Praxis.* 1981; 70:359.

58. Ronningen, H. and Langeland, N. Indomethacin treatment in osteoarthritis of the hip joint. *Acta Orthopedica Scandanavia.* 1979; 50:169-174.

59. Akil, M., Amos, R.S., and Stewart, P. Infertility may sometimes be associated with NSAID consumption. *British Journal of Rheumatism.* 1996; 35:76-78.

60. Wrenn, R. An experimental study of the effect of cortisone on the healing process and tensile strength of tendons. *The Journal of Bone and Joint Surgery.* 1954; 36A:588-601.

61. Truhan, A. Corticosteroids: A review with emphasis on complications of prolonged systemic therapy. *Annals of Allergy.* 1989; 62:375-390.

62. Roenigk, *R. Dermatologic Surgery.* Marcel Dekker, Inc., p. 155.

63. Davis, G. Adverse effects of corticosteroids: 11. *Systemic Clinical Dermatology.* 1986; 4(1):161-169.

64. Gogia, P. Hydrocortisone and exercise effects on articular cartilage in rats. *Archives of Physical Medicine and Rehabilitation.* 1993; 74:463-467.

65. Chandler, G.N. Deleterious effect of intra-articular hydrocortisone. *Lancet.* 1958; 2:661-63.

66. Wiley, R. *Biobalance.* Tacoma, WA: Life Sciences Press, 1989, pp. 7-18.

67. Reams, C. *Choose Life or Death.* Fifth Edition. Tampa, FL: Holistic Laboratories, 1990, pp. 80-85.

68. Wiley, R. *Biobalance.* Tacoma, WA: Life Sciences Press, 1989, pp. 7-18.

69. Sears, B. *The Zone.* New York, NY: Harper Collins Publishers, Inc., 1995.

CHAPTER 6
PROLOTHERAPY, INFLAMMATION, AND HEALING: WHAT'S THE CONNECTION?

1. Robbins, S. *Pathologic Basis of Disease.* Third Edition. Philadelphia, PA: W.B. Saunders Co., 1984, p. 40.

2. Greenfield, B. *Rehabilitation of the Knee: A Problem Solving Approach.* F.A. Davis Co., 1993.

3. Woo, S. Injury and repair of the musculoskeletal soft tissues. *American Academy of Orthopedic Surgeons.* 1987.

4. Mankin, H. Localization of tritiated thymidine in articular cartilage of rabbits inhibits growth in immature cartilage. *Journal of Bone & Joint Surgery.* 1962; 44A:682.

5. Robbins, S. *Pathologic Basis of Disease.* Third Edition. Philadelphia, PA: W.B. Saunders Co., 1984, p. 40.

6. Greenfield, B. *Rehabilitation of the Knee: A Problem Solving Approach.* F.A. Davis Co., 1993.

7. Woo, S. Injury and repair of the musculoskeletal soft tissues. *American Academy of Orthopedic Surgeons.* 1987.

8. Benedetti, R. Clinical results of simultaneous adjacent interdigital neurectomy in the foot. Foot *Ankle International.* 1996; 17:264-268.

CHAPTER 7
PROLO YOUR BACK PAIN AWAY

1. Boden, S. Abnormal magnetic-resonance scans of the lumbar spine in asymptomatic subjects. *The Journal of Bone and Joint Surgery.* 1990; 72A:403-408.

2. Jensen, M. Magnetic resonance imaging of the lumbar spine in people without back pain. *The New England Journal of Medicine.* 1994; 331:69-73.

3. Boden, S. Abnormal magnetic-resonance scans of the lumbar spine in asymptomatic subjects. *The Journal of Bone and Joint Surgery.* 1990; 72A:403-408.

4. Jensen, M. Magnetic resonance imaging of the lumbar spine in people without back pain. *The New England Journal of Medicine.* 1994; 331:69-73.

5. Hackett, G. Shearing injury to the sacroiliac joint. *The Journal of the International College of Surgeons.* 1954; 22:631-639.

6. Bellamy, N. What do we know about the sacroiliac joint? *Seminars in Arthritis and Rheumatism.* 1983; 12:282-313.

7. Paris, S. Physical signs of instability. *Spine.* 1985; 10:277-279.

8. Hackett, G. Shearing injury to the sacroiliac joint. *The Journal of the International College of Surgeons.* 1954; 22:631-639.

9. Mueller, R. *Anesthesia in Current Surgical Diagnosis and Treatment.* Seventh Edition. Los Altes, CA. 1983, pp. 162-169.

10. Burton, C. Conservative management of low back pain. *Postgraduate Medicine.* 5:168-183.

11. Merriman, J. Prolotherapy versus operative fusion in the treatment of joint instability of the spine and pelvis. *Journal of the International College of Surgeons.* 1964; 42:150-159.

12. Ibid.

13. Maynard, J. Morphological and biomechanical effects of sodium morrhuate on tendons. *Journal of Orthopaedic Research.* 1985; 3:236-248.

14. Turner, J. et al. Patient outcomes after lumbar spinal fusions. *Journal of the American Medical Association.* 1992; 286:907-910.

15. Schwarzer, A. The sacroiliac joint in chronic low back pain. *Spine.* 1995 20:31-37.

16. Adams, R. and Victor, M., ed. *Principles of Neurology*. Fourth Edition. St. Louis, MO: McGraw Hill, 1989, pp. 737-738.

17. Hoffman, G. Spinal arachnoiditis—what is the clinical spectrum? *Spine.* 1983; 8:538-540.

18. Guyer, D. The long-range prognosis of arachnoiditis. *Spine.* 1989; 14:1332-1341.

19. Jackson, A. Does degenerative disease of the lumbar spine cause arachnoiditis? A magnetic resonance study and review of the literature. *The British Journal of Radiology.* 1994; 64:840-847.

20. Guyer, D. The long-range prognosis of arachnoiditis. *Spine.* 1989; 14:1332-1341.

21. U.S. Preventive Services Task Force. Screening for adolescent idiopathic scoliosis. *Journal of the American Medical Association.* 1993; 269:2667-2672.

22. Bradford, D. Adult scoliosis. *Clinical Orthopaedics and Related Research.* 1988; 229:70-86.

23. Gunnoe, B. Adult idiopathic scoliosis. *Orthopaedic Review.* 1990; 19:35-43.

24. Keim, H. Adult scoliosis and its management. *Orthopaedic Review.* 1981; 10:41-48.

25. Winter, R. Pain patterns in adult scoliosis. *Orthopedic Clinics of North America.* 1988; 19:339-345.

CHAPTER 8
PROLO ALL YOUR DEGENERATIVE CONDITIONS AWAY!

1. NIH *Consensus Statement on Total Hip Replacement,* 1994; 12:1-31. Published by the NIH in Kensington, Maryland.

2. Cohen, N. Composition and dynamics of articular cartilage; structure, function and maintaining healthy state. *JOSPT.* 1998; 28:203-215.

3. Saaf, J. Effects of exercise on articular cartilage. *Acta Orthop Scand.* 1950; 20:1-83.

4. Buckwalter, J. Articular cartilage. Part 1: Tissue design and chondrocyte-matrix interactions. *Journal of Bone and Joint Surgery.* 1997; 79A: 600-611.

5. Mow, V. *Structure-function relationships for articular cartilage and effects of joint instability and trauma on cartilage function.*

6. Mow, V. *Structure-function relationships for articular cartilage and effects of joint instability and trauma on cartilage function.*

7. Brandt, K. (ed.) Cartilage Changes in Osteoarthritis, pp. 22-42. Indianapolis, IN: *Indiana University School of Medicine Press,* 1990.

8. Mow, V. *Structure-function relationships for articular cartilage and effects of joint instability and trauma on cartilage function.*

9. Mow, V. *Structure-function relationships for articular cartilage and effects of joint instability and trauma on cartilage function.*

10. Mankin, H. The articular cartilages: a review. In *American Academy of Orthopaedic Surgeons: Instructional course lectures, vol. 19,* St. Louis, MO., C.V. Mosby, 1970.

11. Stockwell, R. The cell density of human articular cartilage and costal cartilage. *Journal of Anatomy.* 1967; 101:753.

12. Crelin, E. Changes induced by sustained pressure in the knee joint articular cartilage of adult rabbits. *Anat. Rec.* 1964; 149:113.

13. Mankin, H. Biochemical and metabolic abnormalities in articular cartilage from osteoarthritic human hips. *Journal of Bone and Joint Surgery.* 1970; 52A:424.

14. Mankin, H. The response of articular cartilage to mechanical injury. *Journal of Bone and Joint Surgery.* 1982; 64A:460.

15. Hunter, L. *Rehabilitation of the Injured Knee.* St. Louis, MO: C.V. Mosby, 1984, 149-209.

16. Mankin, H. The response of articular cartilage to mechanical injury. *Journal of Bone and Joint Surgery.* 1982; 64A:460.

17. Mankin, H. The reaction of articular cartilage to injury and osteoarthritis (first of two parts). *New England Journal of Medicine.* 1974; 291:1285.

18. Mankin, H. The reaction of articular cartilage to injury and osteoarthritis (second of two parts). *New England Journal of Medicine.* 1974; 291:1335.

19. Ingman, A. Variations of collagenous and noncollagenous proteins of human knee joint menisci with age and degeneration. *Gerontologia.* 1074; 86:245-252.

20. Arnoczky, S. Meniscus. In *Injury and Repair of the Musculoskeletal Soft Tissues.* Edited by Woo, S. published by the American Academy of Orthopaedic Surgeons, Park Ridge, IL 1987, pp. 487-537.

21. Clark, C. Development of the menisci of the human knee joint. *Journal of Bone and Joint Surgery.* 1983; 65A:538-547.

22. Bessette, G. The Meniscus. *Orthopaedics.* 1992; 15:35-42.

23. Shrive, N. Load-bearing in the knee joint. *Clinical Orthopaedics.* 1978; 131:279-287.

24. Radin, E. Role of menisci in the distribution of stress in the knee. *Clinical Orthopaedics.* 1984; 185:290-294.

25. Ahmed, A. In vitro measurements of the static pressure distribution in synovial joints. Part 1: tibial surface of the knee. *Journal of Biomechanical Engineering.* 1983; 105:216-225.

26. Baratz, M. Meniscal tears: the effect of meniscectomy and of repair on intraarticular contact areas and stress in the human knee. *American Journal of Sports Medicine.* 1986: 14:270-275.

27. Bessette, G. The Meniscus. *Orthopaedics.* 1992; 15:35-42.

28. Radin, E. Role of the menisci in the distribution of stress in the knee. *Clinical Orthopaedics.* 1984; 185:290-294.

29. Seedhom, B. Transmission of the load in the knee joint with special reference to the role of the menisci. *Eng. Med.* 1979: 8:220-228.

30. Bessette, G. The Meniscus. *Orthopaedics.* 1992; 15:35-42.

31. Dandy, D. The diagnosis of problems after meniscectomy. *Journal of Bone and Joint Surgery.* 1975; 57B:349-352.

32. Dandy, D. The diagnosis of problems after meniscectomy. *Journal of Bone and Joint Surgery.* 1975; 57B:349-352.

33. Maletius, W. The effect of partial meniscectomy on the long-term prognosis of knees with localized, severe chondral damage. *The American Journal of Sports Medicine.* 1996; 24:258-262.

34. Bolano, L. Isolated arthroscopic partial meniscectomy. *The American Journal of Sports Medicine.* 1993; 21:432-437.

35. Schmid, A. and Schmid, F. Results after cartilage shaving studied by electron microscopy. *American Journal of Sports Medicine.* 1987; 15:386-387.

36. Salter, R. The effects of continuous compression on living articular cartilage. An experimental investigation. *Journal of Bone and Joint Surgery.* 1960; 42A: 31.

37. Salter, R. The pathological changes in articular cartilage associated with persistent joint deformity: An experimental investigation. In Gordon, D. (ed.) *Studies of Rheumatoid Disease: Proceedings of the Third Canadian Conference on Research in the Rheumatic Diseases.* Toronto, University of Toronto Press, 1965, p. 33.

38. Salter, R. The pathological changes in articular cartilage associated with persistent joint deformity: An experimental investigation. In Gordon, D. (ed.) *Studies of Rheumatoid Disease: Proceedings of the Third Canadian Conference on Research in the Rheumatic Diseases.* Toronto, University of Toronto Press, 1965, p. 33.

39. Salter, R. The effects of continuous compression on living articular cartilage. An experimental investigation. *Journal of Bone and Joint Surgery.* 1960; 42A: 31.

40. Salter, R. The pathological changes in articular cartilage associated with persistent joint deformity: An experimental investigation. In Gordon, D. (ed.) *Studies of Rheumatoid Disease: Proceedings of the Third Canadian Conference on Research in the Rheumatic Diseases.* Toronto, University of Toronto Press, 1965, p. 33.

41. Kuettner, K. *Articular Cartilage and Osteoarthritis.* New York, NY: Raven Press, 1992.

42. Salter, R. The biological concept of continuous passive motion of synovial joints. *Clinical Orthopaedics and Related Research.* 1989; 242: 12-25

43. Salter, R. The effects of continuous compression on living articular cartilage. An experimental investigation. *Journal of Bone and Joint Surgery.* 1960; 42A: 31.

44. Salter, R. Continuous passive motion and the repair of full-thickness defects—a one year follow-up (abstract). *Orthop. Trans.* 1982; 6:266.

45. Salter, R. The healing of intraarticular fractures with continuous passive motion. In Copper R. (ed.) *AAOS Instructional Course Lectures.* St. Louis, MO., C.V. Mosby. 1979.

46. Palmoski, M. Effects of some nonsteroidal anti-inflammatory drugs on proteoglycan metabolism and organization in canine articular cartilage. *Arthritis & Rheumatism.* 1980; 23:1010-1020.

163

47. Salter, R. The biologic concept of continuous passive motion of synovial joints. *Clinical Orthopaedics and Related Research.* 1989; 242: 12-25.

48. Newton, P. The effect of lifelong exercise on canine articular cartilage. *The American Journal of Sports Medicine.* 1997; 25:282-287.

49. Tornkvist, H. Effect of ibuprofen and indomethacin on bone metabolism reflected in bone strength. *Clinical Orthopedics.* 1984; 187:225.

50. Lindholm, T. Ibuprofen effect on bone formation and calcification exerted by the anti-inflammatory drug ibuprofen. *Scandinavian Journal of Rheumatology.* 1981; 10:38.

51. Williams, R. Ibuprofen: An inhibitor of alveolar bone resorption in beagles. *J Periodont Res.* 1988; 23:225.

52. Tornkvist, H. Effect of ibuprofen and indomethacin on bone metabolism reflected in bone strength. *Clinical Orthopedics.* 1984; 187:225.

53. Obeid, G. Effect of ibuprofen on the healing and remodeling of bone and articular cartilage in the rabbit temporomandibular joint. *Journal of Maxillofacial Surgery.* 1992; pp. 843-849.

54. Brandt, K. The effects of salicylates and other nonsteroidal anti-inflammatory drugs on articular cartilage. *American Journal of Medicine.* 1984; 77:65-69.

55. Palmoski, M. Effects of some nonsteroidal anti-inflammatory drugs on proteoglycan metabolism and organization in canine articular cartilage. *Arthritis & Rheumatism.* 1980; 23:1010-1020.

56. Palmoski, M. Effect of salicylate on proteoglycan metabolism in normal canine articular cartilage in vitro. *Arthritis & Rheumatism.* 1979; 22:746-754.

57. Palmoski, M. Marked suppression by salicylate of the augmented proteoglycan synthesis in osteoarthritic cartilage. *Arthritis & Rheumatism.* 1980; 23;83-91.

58. Hugenberg, S. Suppression by nonsteroidal anti-inflammatory drugs on proteoglycan synthesis in articular cartilage. *Arthritis & Rheumatism.* 1992; 35:R29.

59. Brandt, K. Should osteoarthritis be treated with nonsteroidal anti-inflammatory drugs? *Rheumatic Disease Clinics of North America.* 1993; 19:697-712.

60. Palmoski, M. In vitro effect of aspirin on canine osteoarthritic cartilage. *Arthritis & Rheumatism.* 1983; 26:994-1001.

61. Palmoski, M. Marked suppression by salicylate of the augmented proteoglycan synthesis in osteoarthritic cartilage. *Arthritis & Rheumatism.* 1980; 23;83-91.

62. Coke, H. Long term indomethacin therapy of coxarthrosis. *Annals of Rheumatic Diseases.* 1967; 26:346-347.

63. Solomon, L. Drug-induced arthropathy and neurosis of the femoral head. *Journal of Bone and Joint Surgery* (Br). 1973; 55:246-261.

64. Newman, N. Acetabular bone destruction related to nonsteroidal anti-inflammatory drugs. *Lancet.* 1985; 2:11-14.

65. Rashad, S. Effects of nonsteroidal anti-inflammatory drugs on the course of osteoarthritis. *Lancet.* 1989; 2:519-522.

66. Wrenn, R. An experimental study on the effect of cortisone on the healing process and tensile strength of tendons. *The Journal of Bone and Joint Surgery.* 1954; 36A; 588-601.

67. Truhan, A. Corticosteroids: A review with emphasis on complication of prolonged systemic therapy. *Annals of Allergy.* 1989; 62;375-390.

68. Roenigk, R. *Dermatologic Surgery.* Marcel Dekker, Inc., p. 155.

69. Davis, G. Adverse effects of corticosteroids. *Systemic Clinical Dermatology.* 1986; 4:161-169.

70. Gogia, P. Hydrocortisone and exercise effects on articular cartilage in rats. *Archives of Physical Medicine and Rehabilitation.* 1993; 74:463-467.

71. Chandler, G. Deleterious effect of intra-articular hydrocortisone. *Lancet.* 1958; 2:661-663.

72. Chunekamrai, S. Changes in articular cartilage after intra-articular injections of methylprednisolone acetate in horses. *American Journal of Veterinary Research.* 1989; 50:1733-1741.

73. Chunekamrai, S. Changes in articular cartilage after intra-articular injections of methylprednisolone acetate in horses. *American Journal of Veterinary Research.* 1989; 50:1733-1741.

74. Pool, R. Corticosteroid therapy in common joint and tendon injuries of the horse: effect on joints. *Proceedings of the American Association of Equine Practice.* 1980; 26:397-406.

75. From personal correspondence between the author and Michael Herron, D.V.M.

76. Behrens, F. Alteration of rabbit articular cartilage of intra-articular injections of glucocorticoids. *Journal of Bone and Joint Surgery.* 1975; 57A:70-76.

77. Behrens, F. Alteration of rabbit articular cartilage of intra-articular injections of glucocorticoids. *Journal of Bone and Joint Surgery.* 1975; 57A:70-76.

78. Eklhom, R. On the relationship between articular changes and function. *Acta Orthop Scan.* 1951; 21:81-98.

79. Lanier, R. Effects of exercise on the knee joints of inbred mice. *Anat. Rec.* 1946; 94:311-319.

80. Saaf, J. Effects of exercise on articular cartilage. *Acta Orthop Scand.* 1950; 20:1-83.

81. Gogia, P. Hydrocortisone and exercise effects on articular cartilage in rats. *Archives of Physical Medicine and Rehabilitation.* 1993; 74: 463-467.

CHAPTER 9
CONNECTIVE TISSUE DEFICIENCY: THE UNDERLYING CULPRIT IN CHRONIC PAIN AND SPORTS INJURY

1. Mankin, H. The response of articular cartilage to mechanical injury. *Journal of Bone and Joint Surgery.* 1982; 64A: 460.

2. Mankin, H. The reaction of articular cartilage to injury and osteoarthritis (first of two parts). *New England Journal of Medicine.* 1974; 291: 1285.

3. Mankin, H. The reaction of articular cartilage to injury and osteoarthritis (second of two parts). *New England Journal of Medicine.* 1974; 291: 1335.

4. Akenson, W. The chemical basis of tissue repair. In Hunter, L. (ed.) *Rehabilitation of the Injured Knee.* St. Louis, MO: C. V. Mosby Company, 1984, pp. 93-148.

5. Bucci, L. *Nutrition Applied to Injury Rehabilitation and Sports Medicine.* Boca Raton, FL: CRC Press, 1995, pp. 1-20.

6. Whiteside, P. Men's and women's injuries in comparable sports. *The Physician and Sports Medicine.* 1980; 8: 131-140.

7. Liu, S. Estrogen affects the cellular metabolism of the anterior cruciate ligament. A potential explanation for female athletic injury. *The American Journal of Sports Medicine.* 1998; 23: 694-701.

8. Ho, K. Impact of short-term estrogen administration on growth hormone secretion and action: distinct route-dependent effects on connective and bone tissue metabolism. *Journal of Bone and Mineral Research.* 1992; 7: 821-827.

9. Fischer, G. Comparison of collagen dynamics in different tissues under the influence of estradiol. *Endocrinology.* 1972; 93: 1216-1218.

10. Fischer, G. Effect of sex hormones on blood pressure and vascular connective tissue in castrated and noncastrated male rats. *American Journal of Physiology.* 1977; 232: H617-H621.

11. Halme, J. Effect of progesterone on collagen breakdown and tissue collagenolytic activity in the involuting rat uterus. *Journal of Endocrinology.* 1975; 66: 357-362.

12. Lobo, R. Depo-medroxy-progesterone acetate compared with conjugated estrogens for treatment of postmenopausal women. *Obstet Gynecol.* 1984; 66: 789-792.

13. Erlick, Y. Effect of megestrol acetate on flushing and bone metabolism in postmenopausal women. *Maturitas.* 1981; 3: 167-172.

14. Mandel, F. Effect of progestins on bone metabolism in postmenopausal women. *Journal of Reproductive Medicine.* 1982; 27: 511-514.

15. Prior, J. Progesterone as a bone-trophic hormone. *Endocrinology Reviews.* 1990; 11: 386-398.

16. Boik, J. Cancer and Natural Medicine. Princeton, MN: *Oregon Medical Press,* 1996; 43-64.

17. Bone, K. The story of stinging nettles. *In Nutrition and Healing.* 1999; February: 3-4.

18. Dean, W. Hormone replacement alternatives for women. *New Horizons.* 1999; Spring: 1-7.

19. Morales, A. Effects of replacement dose of dehydroepiandrosterone in men and women of advancing age. *The Journal of Clinical Endocrinology and Metabolism.* 1994; 78: 1360-1367.

20. Gaby, A. Dehydroepiandrosterone: Biological Effects and Clinical Significance. *Alternative Medicine Review.* 1996; 1: 60-68.

21. Savvas, M. Type III collagen content in the skin of postmenopausal women receiving estradiol and testosterone implants. *British Journal of Obstetrics and Gynecology.* 1993; 100: 154-156

22. Hall, J. Gonadotropins and the Gonad. In DeGroot, L. (ed.) *Endocrinology.* Philadelphia, PA: W.B. Saunders, 1995, 242-258.

23. Raben, A. Serum sex hormones and endurance performance after a lacto-ovo vegetarian and a mixed diet. *Med Sci Sports Exerc.* 1992; 24: 1290-1297.

24. Guyton, A. (ed.) *Textbook of Medical Physiology.* Philadelphia, PA: W. B. Saunders Company, 1996, 933-944.

25. Erickson, E. Growth hormone and Insulin-like growth factors as anabolic therapies for osteoporosis. *Hormone Research.* 1993; 40: 95-98.

26. Falanga, V. Growth factors and wound healing. *Dermatologic Clinics.* 1993; 11: 66-75

27. Rechler, M. Identification of a receptor for somatomedin-like polypeptide in human fibroblasts. *J Clin Endocrinol Metab.* 1977; 44: 820-827.

28. Bennett, A. Characterization of insulin-like growth factor 1 receptors on cultured rat bone cells: regulation of receptor concentration by glucocorticoids. *Endocrinology.* 1984; 1215: 1577-1583.

29. Cook, J. Mitogenic effects of growth hormone in cultured human fibroblasts. *J Clin Invest.* 1988; 81: 206-212.

30. Hock, J. Insulin-like growth factor 1 has independent effects on bone matrix formation and cell replication. *Endocrinology.* 1988; 122: 254-260.

31. Ho, K. Impact of short-term estrogen administration on growth hormone secretion and action: distinct route-dependent effects on connective and bone tissue metabolism. *Journal of Bone and Mineral Research.* 1992; 7: 821-827.

32. Daughaday, W. Growth hormone, insulin-like growth factors and acromegaly. In Degroot, L. (ed.) *Endocrinology.* Philadelphia, PA: W.B. Saunders, 1995, 303-329.

33. Hall, J. Gonadotropins and the Gonad. In DeGroot, L. (ed.) *Endocrinology.* Philadelphia, PA: W. B. Saunders, 1995, 933-944.

34. Klatz, R. *Grow Young with HGH.* New York City, NY: HarperCollins Publisher, 1997.

APPENDIX A

NUTRITION AND CHRONIC PAIN

1. Reams, C. *Choose Life or Death.* Fifth Edition. Tampa, FL: Holistic Laboratories, 1990, pp. 80-85.

2. D'Adamo, Peter. *Eat Right for Your Type.* New York, NY: G.P. Putnam's Sons, 1996.

3. Wiley, R. *Biobalance.* Tacoma, WA: Life Sciences Press, 1989, pp. 7-18.

APPENDIX B
NEURAL THERAPY
1. Klinghardt, D. Neural Therapy. *Townsend Letter for Doctors and Patients.* July 1995; pp. 96-98.
2. Dosch, P. *Facts about Neural Therapy.* First English Edition. Heidelberg, Germany: Haug Publishers, 1985, pp. 25-30.
3. Dosch, P. *Manual of Neural Therapy.* First English Edition. Heidelberg, Germany: Haug Publishers, 1984, pp. 74-77.
4. Ibid.
5. Dosch, P. *Illustrated Atlas of the Techniques of Neural Therapy with Local Anesthetics.* First English Edition. Heidelberg, Germany: Haug Publishers, 1985.

APPENDIX F
INSURANCE REIMBURSEMENT LETTERS
1. Capen, Karen. "Courts, licensing bodies turning their attention to alternative therapies." *Canadian Medical Associates Journal.* 1996; 156(9): 1307-1308.
2. Joel M. Greene vs. Uniform Medical Plan, June 8, 1992.

APPENDIX G
BEULAH LAND NATURAL MEDICINE CLINIC
1. *The Holy Bible*, New International Version, Revelation 21:27.
1. *The Holy Bible*, New International Version, Matthew 4:23.

INDEX

Beulah Land Press is pleased to offer these books on Prolotherapy written by Dr. Ross and Marion Hauser.

- *Prolo Your Pain Away!* Curing Chronic Pain with Prolotherapy
- *Prolo Your Sports Injuries Away!*
  Curing Sports Injuries and Enhancing Athletic Performance with Prolotherapy
- *Prolo Your Arthritis Pain Away!*
  Curing Disfiguring and Disabling Arthritis Pain with Prolotherapy
- *Prolo Your Back Pain Away!*
  Curing Chronic Back Pain with Prolotherapy
- *Prolo Your Headache and Neck Pain Away!*
  Curing Migraines and Neck Pain with Prolotherapy.
- *Prolo Your Fibromyalgia Pain Away!*
  Curing Disabling Body Pain with Prolotherapy
- *Ligament and Tendon Relaxation Treated by Prolotherapy*
  By George S. Hackett, MD, Gustav A. Hemwall, MD, and Gerald A. Montgomery, MD.

ABOUT THESE BOOKS:

Prolo Your Pain Away!

Read the book that has changed chronic pain management forever. "This is the best book ever written about Prolotherapy, " says Robert C. Atkins, MD, best-selling author of *New Diet Revolution* and medical director of the Atkins Center for Complementary Medicine in New York City, NY. *Prolo Your Pain Away!* details in common lay language the conditions that can be cured with Prolotherapy including arthritis, back pain, migraines, neck pain, Fibromyalgia, spastic torticollis, osteoporosis fracture pain, cancer pain, whiplash, sports injuries, loose joints, TMJ, tendonitis, sciatica, herniated discs, and more! Find out why C. Evertt Koop, MD, former Surgeon General of the United States, a former chronic pain sufferer who was cured by Prolotherapy, says *Prolo Your Pain Away!* is a must-read for anyone experiencing chronic musculoskeletal pain.

Prolo Your Sports Injuries Away!

Just as the original book *Prolo Your Pain Away!* affected the pain management field, *Prolo Your Sports Injuries Away!* has rattled the sports world. Learn the twenty myths of sports medicine including the myths of anti-inflammatory medications; why cortisone shots actually weaken tissue; how ice, rest, and immobilization may actually hurt the athlete; why the common practice of taping and bracing do not stabilize injured areas; and why the arthroscope is one of athletes' worst nightmares!

Did you ever wonder why most career runners and athletes end up with arthritis? This book will explain why this happens and how you can prevent it from happening to you! Prolotherapy is an athlete's best friend because it addresses the root cause of most sports injuries, ligament and tendon weakness. By stimulating the body to repair the painful area, Prolotherapy can make an injured area stronger than its original, uninjured counterpart! Athletes around the country are hailing Prolotherapy as the treatment that not only added more years to their career, but also gave them that additional edge by enhancing their athletic performance. You will learn why Prolotherapy has become the sports medicine treatment of the future and why athletes around the country are curing their sports injuries and enhancing their athletic performance with Prolotherapy.

Prolo Your Arthritis Pain Away!

Studies estimate that 40 million people in the United States suffer from some form of arthritis. By the year 2020 that number will be nearly 60 million. The traditional treatments of arthritis involve anti-inflammatory medication, cortisone shots, and joint replacement surgery. People are often left with the diagnosis "there is nothing else we can do for you." Nothing could be further from the truth. What most people do not realize is that arthritis forms because of an underlying ligament and joint weakness problem. The body responds to this weakness by overgrowing bony formations in the unstable areas, hoping to provide some stabilization to the weak joint. Unfortunately, this is not only painful, but often disfiguring.

Prolotherapy is the best technique available to stimulate the body to strengthen the joint and surrounding ligaments naturally. By doing this, the arthritis process stops and the pain can be eliminated. This book will detail why arthritis sufferers around the country are throwing away the anti-inflammatory medications and returning to the activities that they used to enjoy. Prolotherapy has given life back to many arthritis sufferers. Gone are the days of waking up feeling stiff and sore.

Prolo Your Back Pain Away!

Stan Mikita, former Chicago Black Hawk Hockey star and hall-of-famer, was about to cut a magnificent career short because of a back injury. Six weeks prior to the 1971-1972 season opening, Mr. Mikita could not even get out of bed because of severe sciatica and back pain. He found Prolotherapy as a treatment option that got him back on his skates again. Learn why Stan enthusiastically says, "Prolotherapy definitely extended my NHL career eight years and gave me complete relief of my back pain!" Learn why MRI scans may erroneously diagnose "disc problems" forcing people into unnecessary surgeries. Prolotherapy can help the painful conditions such as degenerated disc disease, sciatica, arthritis, spinal stenosis, and even herniated discs. This is why people with chronic back pain are saying "no" to surgery and "yes" to Prolotherapy!

Prolo Your Headache and Neck Pain Away!

Years ago, it was going to be another ruined evening for the Hausers. Marion had another migraine headache. She finally decided try Prolotherapy and put an end of the suffering. Boy, is she glad that she did! You will also be glad if you suffer from migraines, tension, or cluster headaches. Marion went from being a skeptic to someone who now writes books on the topic! Prolotherapy stimulates the body to repair painful areas. Don't most headaches start out with neck or shoulder pain? Learn about a lesser-known syndrome called Barré-Lieou Syndrome, which is one of the most common causes of headaches. Some of the associated symptoms include ringing in the ears, sinus pressure, dizziness, and neck pain. Ligament injury in the neck is usually the cause of head forward posture, which leads to chronic neck pain and headaches. Prolotherapy causes the vertebrae in the neck to stay in alignment. Good alignment means good posture. Good posture means fewer headaches. No more headaches mean good-bye to pain pills. Learn why many former headache sufferers found hope with Prolotherapy.

Prolo Your Fibromyalgia Pain Away!

An epidemic number of people in the United States wake up in the morning feeling tired, sore, and achy. Upon physical examination, tender points are found all over the body. Women may be given the concurrent diagnoses of migraine headaches and endometriosis. They are told to exercise and take antidepressant medication. Nothing can be done to cure the problem... until now. Learn why over 90 percent of Fibromyalgia sufferers respond well to Prolotherapy. People with Fibromyalgia often suffer from fungus infections that have a tremendously detrimental effect on soft tissue formation, including the ligaments and tendons. Treatment of this fungus, in conjunction with Prolotherapy, has given hope to many suffering from the often debilitating Fibromyalgia.

Ligament and Tendon Relaxation Treated by Prolotherapy

After performing Prolotherapy for over 40 years, the world's most experienced Prolotherapist, Gustav A. Hemwall, MD, died at the age of 90. His legacy and experience are preserved in this 5TH edition of the book written by the originator himself, George S. Hackett, MD. Dr. Hackett wrote many of the words in this book. This book was written to demonstrate the technique of Prolotherapy to physicians. Many case studies are also presented. Much of what is known about Prolotherapy comes from the authors of this book.

PURCHASING INFORMATION:
1-800-RX-PROLO
1-800-797-7656
www.caringmedical.com and   www.proloinfo.com

FOR FURTHER INFORMATION:
Beulah Land Press • 715 Lake St., Suite 600 • Oak Park, IL 60301
E-Mail: drhauser@caringmedical.com

Would you like to become a patient? We have a national referral base and see patients from all over the country. Dr. Ross Hauser and Dr. Nicole King are two of the country's most experienced clinicians in Prolotherapy and other natural medicine techniques. Caring Medical is a comprehensive natural medicine center only minutes from downtown Chicago in the beautiful suburb of Oak Park, Illinois. The center is only 30 minutes from either O'Hare or Midway airports.

Besides Prolotherapy, the center also offers:

- Metabolic Typing
- Anti-aging Regimes (including biological aging measurement)
- Chelation Therapy
- Natural Hormone Replacement
- Nutritional/herbal Counseling
- Ozone Therapy
- Neural Therapy
- Photoluminescence
- Other specific regimes to reverse connective tissue deficiency

Caring Medical services clients with every human disease including chronic pain, rheumatologic diseases, chronic fatigue, cancer, diabetes, high blood pressure, digestive and heart conditions, as well as other chronic disabling diseases.

CARING MEDICAL BELIEVES THE CARE OF THE PATIENT BEGINS WITH CARING.

To learn more about the life-changing natural medicine regimes at Caring Medical, you can contact our office in one of the following ways:

CONTACT OUR OAK PARK OFFICE AT:

Caring Medical and Rehabilitation Services
715 Lake St., Suite 600 • Oak Park, IL 60301
PH.: 708-848-7789 • FAX: 708-848-7763
URL: www.caringmedical.com
E-MAIL: drhauser@caringmedical.com

FOR MORE INFORMATION